Neuromuscular block

Stanley Feldman FRCA

*Professor Emeritus, Magill Department
of Anaesthetics, University of London;
Honorary Consultant, Chelsea and
Westminster Hospital, London, UK*

BUTTERWORTH
HEINEMANN

1996

Butterworth-Heinemann
Linacre House, Jordan Hill, Oxford OX2 8DP
A division of Reed Educational & Professional Publishing Ltd

⬲ A member of the Reed Elsevier plc group

OXFORD BOSTON JOHANNESBURG
MELBOURNE NEW DELHI SINGAPORE

First published 1996

British Library Cataloguing in Publication Data
Feldman, Stanley A.
  Neuromuscular Block
  I. Title
  615.781

ISBN 0 7506 1764 0

Library of Congress Cataloguing in Publication Data
Feldman, Stanley A.
  Neuromuscular block/Stanley Feldman.
  p. cm.
  Includes bibliographical references and index.
  ISBN 0 7506 1764 0
  1. Neuromuscular blocking agents. I. Title.
  RM312.F443 1996   95-45603
  615'.773—dc20   CIP

Typeset by BC Typesetting, Bristol
Printed and bound by Hartnolls Ltd, Bodmin, Cornwall

Contents

Preface

'Academia should encourage debate on established thought. It should strip away covering veneer of certainty and lay bare illusion.'

The story is told that at a graduation ceremony in a south-western University in the USA the Dean congratulated the successful students on passing their examinations but he cautioned: 'In 10–15 years time we expect to discover that half of what you have learnt is either wrong or misleading – the trouble is, we do not know which half!'

This book has been written with this aphorism in mind. There is no doubt that part of what is currently taught as the classical pharmacology of neuromuscular block is wrong. It is the duty of teachers to encourage an enquiring and questioning attitude to what is being taught and to point out the many paradoxes that cannot be explained by conventional ideas. It is the task of research to seek the answer to those questions.

In this monograph I have tried to present alternative explanations to address some of these paradoxes but there is no way of knowing whether the answers I propose are as fallible as the ones they replace or modify. As Karl Popper pointed out[1], science evolves by disproof of one theory and the proposal of alternatives. This is essential in a clinical speciality as it is seldom possible to fulfil Koch's postulates of proof. As a result, the casual association of events is frequently taken as evidence of a causal relationship and it is only by questioning these relationships that the true nature of cause and effect be determined. It is also true in science that the Parkinson bicycle-shed phenomenon comes into play[2] – a theory supported by obscure mathematics or a single observation from the cutting edge of molecular science is often more readily accepted than observations made by simple experimental clinical models, as the reader finds it easier to question the logic of simple observations than the results of esoteric experiments on a cell from a primitive animal species using complex research tools. This is not to say that these experiments are inappropriate, but that in some circumstances they can lead to questionable extrapolations when applied to anaesthetized patients.

In this book I have tried to balance the present, too-ready acquiescence with the validity of current hypotheses, with the questions that they fail to address or cannot answer so that the reader is made aware of the uncertainties surrounding presently accepted ideas. The views presented are based on some 35 years of clinical observation and experimentation with neuromuscular blocking drugs. This has led to a concept of how neuromuscular block is produced and how normal transmission is re-established, which offers alternative explanations of experiences that anaesthetists observe every day when using neuromuscular blocking agents. I have drawn heavily upon our own research experience in order to explain these concepts in a manner that is readily understandable to clinical anaesthetists.

This book is not meant to be a definitive textbook on muscle relaxants – there are many excellent texts available on this subject. It emphasizes what is *not* known, and the information that is presented as fact but leaves questions unanswered.

Much is new information; many of the explanations offered are controversial. If it causes readers to realize the limitations of our knowledge it will have served a purpose; if it makes some question established theories it will have succeeded. Formulating the concepts presented in this book has been like trying to guess the pattern of a jigsaw in which several key pieces are missing and a few parts from another puzzle are included. Only time and further experimentation will tell whether the ideas presented are a correct interpretation or whether they too will prove to be wrong.

References

1. Popper K. (1968) *The Logic of Scientific Discovery.* New York: Harper and Row
2. Parkinson CN. (1958) *Parkinson's Law.* London: Monroy

Introduction

I first became interested in the muscle relaxant drugs in 1956 when, under the influence of my teachers, Geoffrey Organe, who introduced C_{10} into clinical anaesthesia, J.B. Wyman, who worked with Bill Paton on C_5 and C_6, and Cyril Scurr, who introduced suxamethonium to the UK, I realized that these drugs did not always behave in a predictable manner. In 1957 I spent a year as research fellow in the University of Washington, Seattle, working with Lucien E. Morris and Evan Frederickson. It was work carried out during that period that convinced me that there were gaps in our understanding of the mechanism of neuromuscular block and its reversal. In 1962 I observed the inability of neostigmine to reverse residual, quite minor paresis following the administration of gallamine to a patient until after haemodolysis, and I realized that this single event could not be explained on the basis of the competition theory alone. Other factors had to play a part. The question was, why did neostigmine not reverse residual neuromuscular block in the presence of a low, subparalytic level of non-depolarizing drug? Much of my research in the past 35 years has been directed to answering this question, which is fundamental to our understanding of how drugs block neuromuscular conduction and how neuromuscular conduction is re-established. Gradually over this time we have accumulated evidence, like a detective with a mystery to solve. We have tested the evidence, we have found corroboration and we have produced what I believe is a likely explanation of the puzzle.

The reader might now better understand why so many of my early experiments were performed using gallamine, a drug hardly used today.

I would like to acknowledge two major influences that have sustained my investigations. The first is due to the friendship and encouragement of a group of researchers who first met at Westminster Hospital in 1975 at the first of the International Muscle Relaxant Meetings. This was the brainchild of David Savage and Sandor Agoston and it introduced me to Bill Bowman, Francis Foldes, Ron Miller, Jan Crul and many other outstanding workers in the field. The second, more recent influence has been my research fellows in the Magill Department of Anaesthetics, Nick Fauvel, Nick Campkin, Jeavon Hood, Adrian England, Imre Redai and Katrina Richards. This last group has helped me accomplish in 5 years what would have taken decades without their enthusiasm.

Like a good detective story, we believe we have identified the cause of the problem I first observed 35 years ago. We have reduced the list of the possible causes of the gallamine effect. It now only remains to pinpoint the actual mechanism by which the effect is produced, before we finally have all the evidence we need to close the investigation.

I would also like to acknowledge especially the help I have had in preparing this manuscript from my wife, Carole, and Miss Simone Bird.

History

It was the writings, in Latin, by the Italian monk Peter Martyr d'Anghera in 1516 that first described the poisoned arrows used by the South American Indians and that brought news of curare to the court of Ferdinand and Elizabeth in Spain and hence to the rest of Europe.[1] He described a concoction into which the arrows were dipped as containing the 'stings of scorpions', the 'heads of deadly ants' and 'the juice they distil from certain trees'. The secret recipe for the manufacture of the poison was restricted to a small number of old women who, he wrote, often died from inhaling the fumes. His account also details cures used by Indians for the ill effects of the poison, including avoidance of 'excessive pleasures of the tables' and 'sexual abstinence for two years'!

However, both his account published in *De Orbe Novo* and that of the Spanish physician Monardes in his *Joyfull Newes out of the Newe Founde Worlde*, which was translated from Latin into English in 1577,[2] retold many anecdotal stories which were often fanciful descriptions, much embellished, to appeal to the imagination of a wondrous and impressionable home audience.

More accurate descriptions of the use of the poisoned arrows occur in the account of Sir Walter Raleigh's visit to Guinea (1594–95).[3] Hakluyt reported on the terrible death of those struck by these arrows.[4] 'They endured a most ugly and lamentable death'. He confirmed that no cure for the death had been obtained in spite of the torture and martyrdom of many Indians. He believed, however, that the priests did have a cure, but only passed it on from father to son. The name *ourari* given to the poison was used by Hakluyt in his accounts in which he describes convulsions and 'the breaking of their bowels' accompanying the terrible effects of the poison.

It is interesting to note that most early reports suggest a convulsive rather than a paralytic death following wounding with the poison. This may well have been due to strychnine contamination of the crude poison as the bark and root of *Nux strychnos* (*Strychnos toxifera*) was frequently incorporated in the lethal cocktail (Fig. 1.1).

It was recognized that not all South American poison arrows contained the same ingredients. This led the German chemist Boehm to the classification of curares according to the means of their preparation. In Equador and Peru the poison was prepared from the bark of the creeper

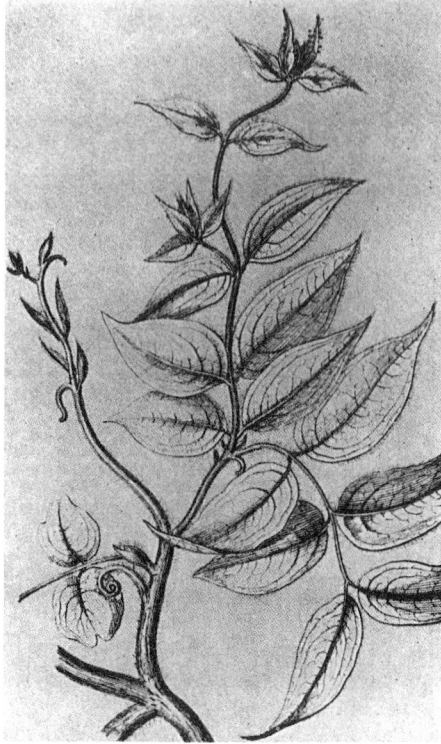

Fig.1.1 Drawing of *Strychnos toxifera* (Bentham collection).

Chondodendron tomentosum (Fig. 1.2) by extracting the juice – a mixture of various alkaloids – and storing it in tubes, whilst in Orinoco and Guyana the extract of *Strychnos toxifera* was often used together with other roots. Since this preparation was stored in gourds it was called gourd, or calabash curare.[5]

It was Charles Waterton's objective and detailed descriptions of the Macoushi Indians of Demerara and Essequibo, published in 1879 in his *Wanderings in South America*,[6] that provided the first scientific account of the action of *wourali*. On his return he persuaded Benjamin Brodie, a British surgeon, to use the drug in experiments on donkeys and chickens. He concluded:

> It affects the nervous system and thus destroys vital functions; it is also said to be harmless provided it does not touch the blood. However, this is certain, when a sufficient quantity of it enters the blood, death is the inevitable consequence; but there is no alteration in the colour of the blood and both the blood and flesh may be eaten with safety.

He gives vivid descriptions of the preparation of the poison from the vine *wourali* and its combination with other glutinous extracts from berries, bushes, red ants and snakes.

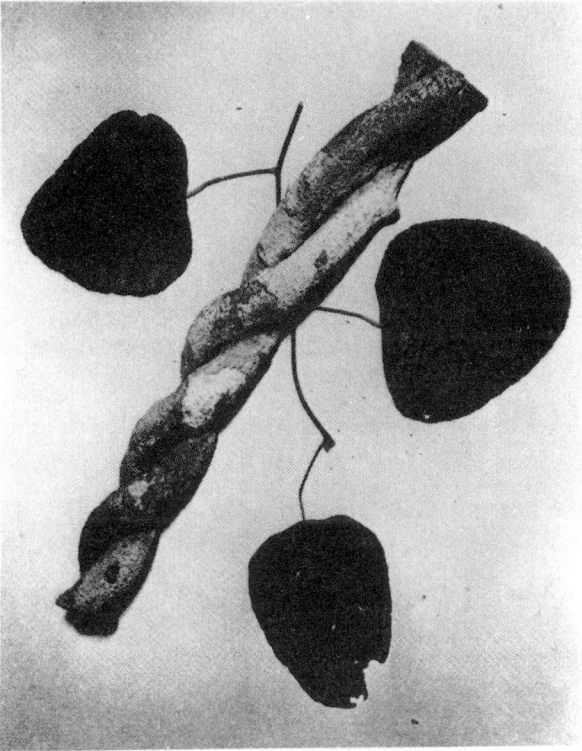

Fig. 1.2 Stem and leaves of *Chondodendron tomentosum.*

The early studies of the South American arrow poison was directed towards finding a cure for its effects and determining whether its fumes were toxic, as had been suggested by early travellers, including de la Condamine, whose account of his travels was published in Paris in 1745.[7] This led the Abbé Felix Fontanna[8] and others in Leiden, Holland, using specimens of the drug obtained from the distinguished British physician Heberden, to expose animals to the fumes produced when the crude extract was heated. They demonstrated that the drug was harmless when inhaled and when taken in food but lethal when injected into flesh.

It was the poison brought back to England by Charles Waterton and given to Dr E.N. Bancroft that was used in the experiments of Benjamin Brodie and reported to the Royal Society in 1811 and 1812.[9,10] Brodie dramatically demonstrated that curare killed by cessation of breathing and that, if the lungs of the animal were artificially ventilated by means of a bellows, life would be preserved. The public demonstration of the total paralysis of a 'she ass' for 2 h, during which time it was kept alive by artificial ventilation using a bellows inserted into the trachea, demonstrated how *wourali* killed its victims. It is reported that the ass lived for many years after this experiment.

However, it was Claude Bernard[11] who finally elucidated the action of the poison on the neuromuscular transmission. His simple, unequivocal experiments were reported in his *Leçons sur les effects des substances toxiques et médicamentueses* published between 1857 and 1866. Bernard used frogs in his experiments and was undoubtedly the first to use an isolated-limb experiment. He tied a ligature around the artery to the hind limb before administering the drug systemically. The result is described in his Leçons 21–25 published in 1856–1866.

> When we poisoned a frog, after ligation of the hind quarters, the toxic action you saw was exerted only on the fore quarters. The reflex movements produced by pinching the skin of the fore quarters demonstrated the integrity of the sensory system. The paralysis therefore bears solely on the motor nerve. . . .
>
> Does the paralysis which has invaded the motor nerves from the periphery to the centre stop at the junction of the anterior and posterior roots or does it extend as far as the spinal cord?[11]

Bernard observed the paralysis of the muscles of the body whilst those in the isolated hind limb remained responsive to stimulation of the nerve (Fig. 1.3). He observed that direct muscle stimulation evoked a response even in the paralysed animal. He concluded that the drug prevented the passage of nerve stimulation to the muscle. However, he believed that the poison acted on the spine or spinal roots of motor nerves. He demonstrated that stimulation of the nerve to the paralysed limb produced movement in the other non-paralysed limb and concluded that the sensory nervous system remained unaffected. He concluded that the action of curare was exclusively upon the motor nervous system. His observations revealed the terrible drama of curare poisoning, with the victim remaining lucid whilst unable to move. Bernard's description is poignant: 'within the still body and staring death like eyes, feeling and intelligence persist strongly. His consciousness persists whilst his organs die one by one, imprisoned within a cadaver'.[11]

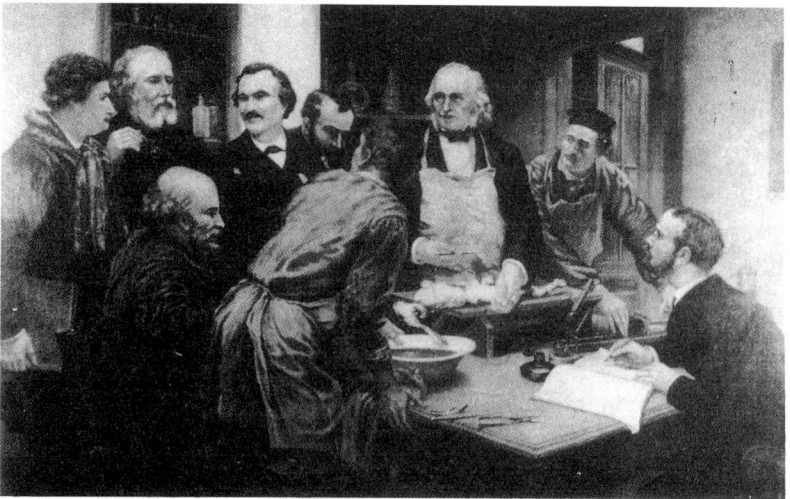

Fig. 1.3 Drawing of Claude Bernard demonstrating to his pupils.

However, Bernard missed the precise implication of his findings, which was left to his pupil Vulpian.[9] Vulpian proposed that curare acted on the neuromuscular junction at the motor end-plate, the morphology of which had recently been described by Kühne.

The final chapter in the story started with the demonstration by Langley of a chemical transmitter nicotine, which caused muscle contraction and which was blocked by curare.[12] In 1921, Otto Loewi[13] demonstrated that a chemical transmitter was produced by vagal stimulation and in 1934 Dale[15] and Dale and Feldberg[15] discovered that acetylcholine was released during neuromuscular transmission and that a close intra-arterial injection of acetylcholine caused muscle contraction. It was then a short step to the demonstration in 1936–37 by Dale and colleagues[16] and by Bacq and Brown[17] that curare blocked this action. The mystery of South American arrow poison was at last solved by the pharmacologists of University College, London.

It was not until the publication in 1942 by Harold Griffith and Enid Johnson of their experience in 25 patients using the curare preparation Intocostrin during cyclopropane and ether anaesthesia that the potential therapeutic usefulness of the arrow poison was eventually established.

There were previous attempts to use crude preparations of curare to treat patients. Spencer Wells, a lecturer in surgery at Grosvenor Place School, used *woorara* in 3 patients who developed postoperative tetanus in 1859; unfortunately, all 3 patients died.[18] However, he did recount that 2 patients had relief of their spasms, although one clearly had difficulty in coughing up her sputum. In his paper, Spencer Wells refers to other cases of tetanus being treated with *woorara*, by Vella in Turin and Manec and Chassaignac in Paris.

In 1869 there is a record of curare being used to treat epilepsy in a man aged 23. As late as 1941 curare was being recommended for the treatment of muscular spasms and convulsive states such as strychnine poisoning, eclampsia and status epilepticus. It is suggested that it was the action in painful muscle spasms that provided the driving force which led Dr Richard Gill to obtain the drug from the Indians in the area of his ranch in Ecuador.[19] In spite of many difficulties, Gill brought samples of the extracts of many different plants to the research laboratories of Squibb in 1948 and it was from these samples that McIntyre of the University of Nebraska extracted the pure curare which was in the samples of Intocostrin supplied to Harold Griffith. Professor McIntyre supplied curare to Professor Bennett in his university; the latter used it successfully to modify the convulsions of metrazol shock therapy.[20]

The Squibb company had the foresight to see the potential for the drug in reducing muscle tone in anaesthesia and originally approached Dr Rovenstein of New York. Having observed the cessation of respiration it produced in a patient anaesthetized by Dr Papper in his hospital, Rovenstein was of the opinion that it would be too dangerous to use in anaesthetized, sick patients because of the paralysis it produced. As a result, it was Dr Griffith and Dr Johnson who first used Intocostrin, refined from the crude extract from Ecuador, during anaesthesia in 25 patients in the Homeopathic Hospital in Montreal.[21] Dr Griffith recognized the early onset of paralysis and intubated and ventilated his patients when this was indicated. It is a salutary comment that Griffith wrote that he would not like to see the widespread use of the drug: 'It should not be used indiscriminately because the inexperienced anaesthetist is too inefficient to obtain muscle relaxation by ordinary procedures'. Unfortunately, his strictures are seldom followed in present-day practice, where muscle relaxants are too often used indiscriminately to cover inadequate anaesthesia and are all too frequently used for operations requiring no muscle relaxation.

References

1. Martyr d'Anghera P. (1516) *De Orbe Novo*. English translation by MacNutt FA. New York: Putnam, 1912
2. Monardes N. (1571) *Joyfull Newes out of the Newe Founde Worlde*. Curare and its Usage. K Bryn Thomas. London: Pitman, 1964
3. Raleigh SW. *The Discovery of the Large, Rich and Beautiful Empire of Guinea* (1596)
4. Hakluyt A. (1598) Relation of the second voyage to Guinea. Curare and its Usage. K Bryn Thomas. London: Pitman, 1964
5. Boehm R. (1886) *Chemische Studien uber das Curare*. Leipzig
6. Waterton C. (1879) *Wanderings in South America*. London: MacMillan
7. de la Condamine F. (1745) *Relation abregée d'un voyage fait dans l'interieur de l'Amerique Meridionale*. Paris: Balliere
8. Fontanna F. Mémoire: sur le poison Americain appeler Ticunas et sur quelques autre poisons vegeteaux. *Mem Acad R Sci* 1745
9. Brodie BC. Experiments and observations on the different modes in which death is produced by certain vegetable poisons. *Phil Trans R Soc Lond* 1811; 194–195
10. Brodie BC. Further experiments and observations on the action of poisons on the animal systems. *Phil Trans R Soc Lond* 1812; 207–209
11. Bernard C. (1856–57) *Leçons sur les effects des substances toxiques et médicamenteuses*. Paris: Baillière
12. Langley JN. On the reaction of cells and of nerve endings to certain poisons, chiefly as regards the reaction of striated muscle to nicotine and to curare. *J Physiol* 1905; **33:** 374–413
13. Loewi O. Uber humorale Ubertragbarkeit der Herenvenwirkung. *Pflugers Archives*. 1921; **189:** 239–246
14. Dale HH. Chemical transmission of effects of nerve impulses. *Br Med J* 1934; **i:** 835–840
15. Dale HH & Feldberg W. Chemical transmission at voluntary nerve endings in muscle. *J Physiol* 1934; **81:** 39–42
16. Dale HH, Feldberg W & Vogt M. Release of acetylcholine at voluntary motor nerve endings. *J Physiol* 1936; **86:** 353–380
17. Bacq ZM & Brown GL. Pharmacological experiments on mammalian voluntary muscle in relation to the theory of chemical transmission. *J Physiol* 1937; **89:** 45–60
18. Wells ST. Three cases of tetanus in which woorara was used. *Proc R Med Chir Soc Lond* 1859; **3:** 142–157
19. Gill RC. Curari, the flying death. *Natural History* 1935; **36:** 279–286
20. Bennett AE. Preventing traumatic complications in convulsive shock therapy by curare. *JAMA* 1940; **144:** 322–324
21. Griffith HR & Johnson GE. The use of curare in general anaesthesia. *Anesthesiology* 1942; **3:** 418–420

2

The neuromuscular junction

The gross morphology of the end-plate region, in which the motor nerve terminates on the surface of the muscle it innervates, was demonstrated by Kühne over 100 years ago.

Since that time the detailed morphology of the region has been described and the physiological importance of the region recognized. Dale and his coworkers working at University College, London in the late 1930s produced overwhelming evidence that the acetylcholine (ACh) which was released at the motor nerve endings[1] acted to amplify and modulate the effect of motor nerve activity upon the muscle. He termed this action nicotinic. The demonstration of specific receptors sensitive to ACh on the postjunctional membrane,[2-4] originally proposed by Langley in 1906,[5,6] and the pharmacological evidence of ACh receptors at the prejunctional motor nerve endings originally proposed by Koelle in 1961[7] and subsequently demonstrated by others,[8-13] has allowed a better understanding of how neuromuscular conduction is controlled. Scientists working in this field have been fortunate to have good, highly specific ligands for the postsynaptic receptors such as α-bungarotoxin from the banded Krait snake (Fig. 2.1) and the presence in nature of large modified end-organs, which demonstrate the potential amplifying power of cholinergic mechanisms, such as the electric organs of the stingray (*Torpedo marmorata*), in which about 50% of the electric organ protein is receptor, and electric eel (*Electropax electrophus*). Unfortunately, no highly specific ligand has been found for the putative presynaptic receptors, nor is there any equivalent large model of a presynaptic receptor available for scrutiny. As a result, our knowledge of the structure of these receptors remains speculative, although it is reasonably assumed that they will prove to be similar to the family of ACh receptors found in ganglia and the central nervous system. These are also pentameric structures but possess only two types of subunits. Despite this, these structures demonstrate a high degree of amino acid sequence homogenicity.[14,15]

The neuromuscular junction

As the motor nerve approaches the muscle it loses its myelin sheath and divides into many fibrils. In focally innervated muscle, nerve fibrils pierce

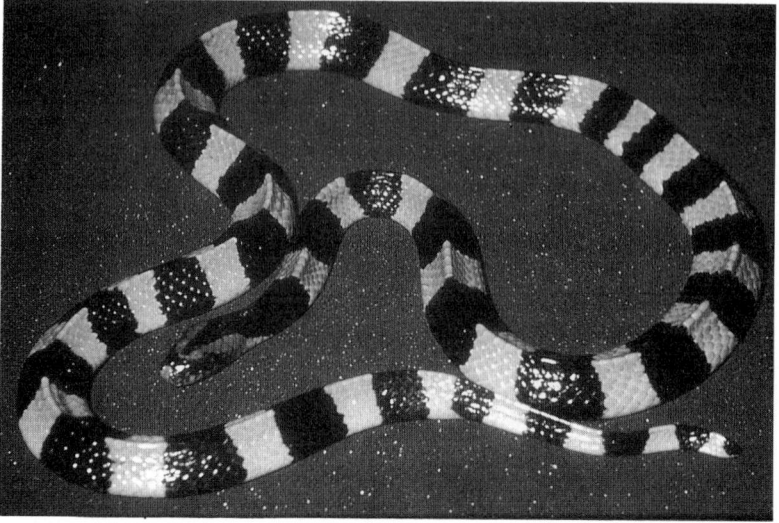

Fig. 2.1 The banded Krait, whose venom is the source of α-bungarotoxin.

the epimysium approximately midway along the belly of the muscle fibre and enter a shallow depression on the surface of the muscle (Fig. 2.2). This primary cleft contains a series of parallel troughs, enfolded upon the muscle to produce narrow deep clefts – the secondary clefts. As nerve fibril pierces the muscle, the neurilemma coating the nerve fuses with the epimysium of the muscle. The nerve ending (presynaptic zone) is separated by a gap of about 60–100 nm from the postsynaptic membrane of the muscle by the synaptic or junctional cleft. The whole structure is enclosed by the tent-like Schwann cell membrane. The cholinoceptors, the structure containing the specific ACh recognition sites (AChR), are densely packed in clusters on the postsynaptic membrane around the mouths of secondary clefts (Fig. 2.3).

The enclosing Schwann cell membrane which separates the synaptic cleft from the extracellular fluid (ECF) appears anatomically to be a continuation of the neurilemma. There is little evidence that this membrane impedes the ingress or egress of water solutes or neuromuscular blocking drugs. It does, however, retain colloid and the formed structural contents of the synaptic cleft and separates them from the extracellular water which bathes the motor end-plate. Water-soluble drugs reach the synaptic cleft and affect the AChR by diffusion from the ECF. It is the concentration of drug in this compartment that influences the magnitude of their effect.

In birds, reptiles and amphibians the muscles may have multiple innervations with two or more end-plates innervated by the same motor nerve fibril. This type of muscle responds differently from focally innervated muscle; it undergoes a continuous contracture in the presence of ACh and agonist drugs. Multiple innervated muscle fibres have been described in the extraocular muscles of the human eye and may be responsible for the raised intraocular pressure observed after suxamethonium as a result of 'squeezing' the orbit. In more primitive species, such as the crustacean

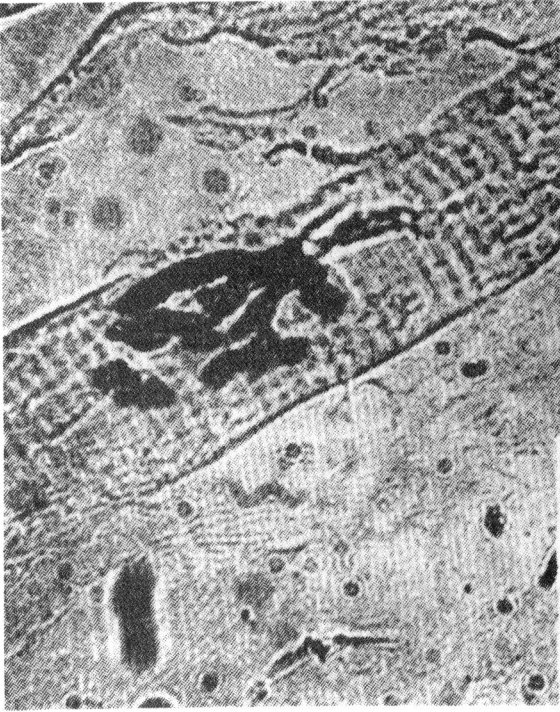

Fig. 2.2 Motor nerve fibrils terminate in shallow gutters on the belly of the muscle fibre. Autoradiograph using H^3 curare.

bivalve, ACh causes a contracture of the adductor muscle without evidence of any neural innervation (this action is responsible for the difficulty one finds in opening oysters!).

All the muscle fibres supplied by one motor nerve, together with the neuron from which the nerve originated, constitute a motor unit. The number of muscle fibres innervated by a single nerve fibre determines the flexibility of the response of which it is capable. As a result, muscles with large numbers of fibres innervated by a single nerve fibre, such as the gastrocnemius and other postural muscles, will not be able to achieve the fine movements that are possible in the lumbrical muscles of the hand, in which the motor unit is one-tenth to one-twentieth of its size.

Focally innervated muscle obeys the 'all-or-none' law. As a result, each fibre will either contract in response to a stimulus or fail to do so. Gradations of muscle contraction are due to the less sensitive muscle fibres within a single muscle failing to respond. Under the usual physiological conditions all the muscle fibres in a motor unit contract together and have similar thresholds of excitability. However, in degenerative conditions this may not occur. It is evident that if one is to measure neuromuscular conduction under differing degrees of block, it is essential to ensure that even the most resistant muscles contract, if possible, in response to a motor nerve stimulus in order to ensure a uniformity of

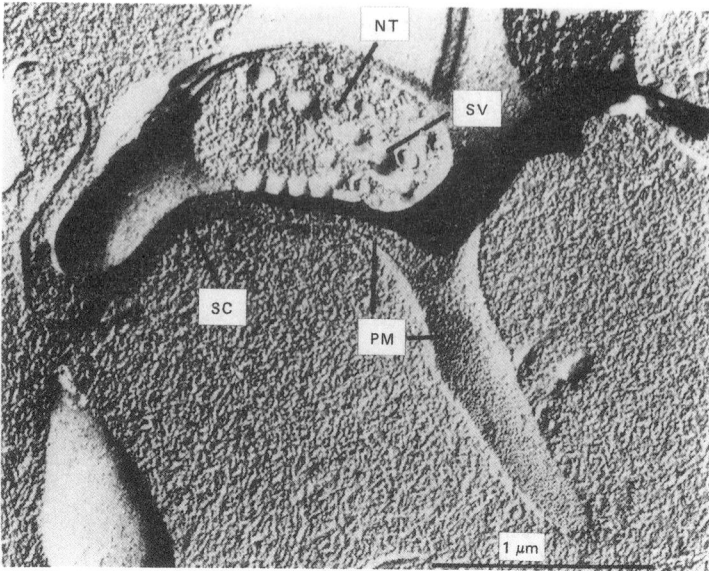

Fig. 2.3 The neuromuscular synapse showing the cut end of the motor nerve (NT) containing synaptic vesicules (SV), the synaptic cleft (SC) and the secondary cleft. The cholinoceptors (PM) are situated on the shoulders of the secondary clefts.

response. For this reason it is necessary to ensure at all times that the stimulus is supramaximal.

The blood supply to the motor end-plate has not been well-studied, although it is of importance in drug delivery to the synapse. The blood vessels accompanying the motor nerve (vasa comitantes) send a branch to the end-plate region and appear to be a reason for the apparent 'luxury perfusion' of this and other synapses (Fig. 2.4). The blood supply to the total muscle varies greatly according to the activity of the muscle but in the resting state, i.e. in the anaesthetized patient when a neuromuscular blocking drug is administered, it would not be anticipated to provide sufficient flow to the end-plate to explain the rapid onset of action of drugs such as suxamethonium.

Microanatomy of the neuromuscular junction

The neuromuscular junction contains the ending of the motor nerve fibril (the presynaptic membrane), the synaptic gap or primary cleft and the secondary clefts produced by the gutters on the muscle seen in cross-section (the postsynaptic membrane; Fig. 2.5). The neuromuscular junction is enclosed by the Schwann cell membrane. The synaptic cleft contains ECF and basement membrane. The basement membrane is composed of crumpled sheets of mucopolysaccharide which, on cross-section, appear as an irregular lattice within which groups of long-tailed molecules of acetylcholinesterase protrude.

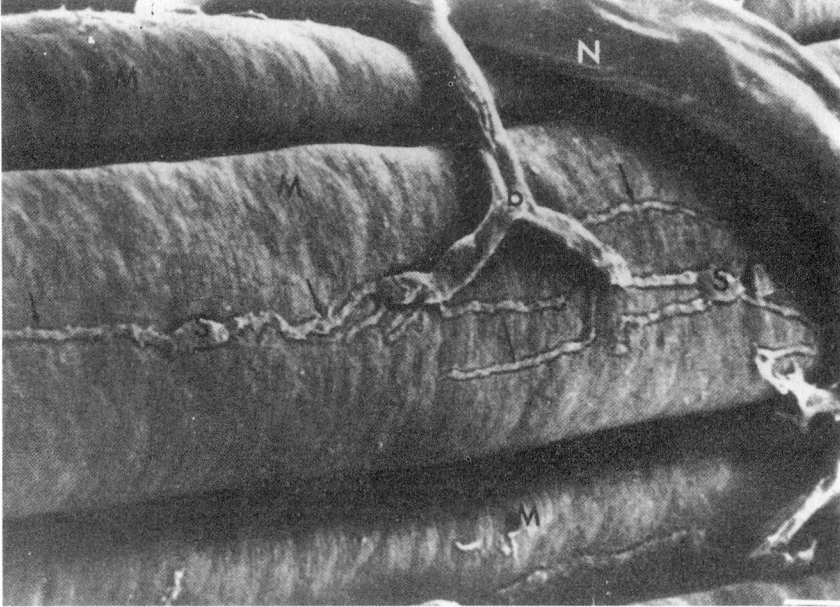

Fig. 2.4 Motor end-plate showing blood supply (b) from a vasa comitantes.

The presynaptic membrane on the nerve terminal is traversed by thickened ridges between which lie the active zones in which the ACh vesicles discharge their contents. The microanatomy of the active zones reveals them as four rows of paired particles, each of which is believed to be a tethering site for an ACh vesicle prior to the discharge of its contents into the synaptic clefts. This zone is closely associated with calcium transport across the presynaptic membrane.[16] The postsynaptic membrane on the muscle is enfolded by the secondary clefts which appear as narrow-necked sacs on cross-section. It is around the mouths of these secondary clefts that the receptor pentamers with their AChR sites are massed. The area is readily stained using gold thioaectate, which indicates the presence of cholinesterase in the substrate.

The cholinoceptor pentamer

Most of our detailed understanding of the cholinoceptor on the post-synaptic membrane relates to studies on the electric organ of *Torpedo marmorata* (the sting ray) and *Electropax electrophus* (electric eel). Studies on isolated receptors have demonstrated that this structure is composed of four distinct subunits, α, β, γ, δ which form the pentamer – the α unit is duplicated (Fig. 2.6). Studies on reconstituted receptors expressed in xenopus oocytes and human embryonic kidney cells have demonstrated that all but the β unit are essential to ensure an ACh response. Patch-clamp experiments have demonstrated that the pentamer responds to

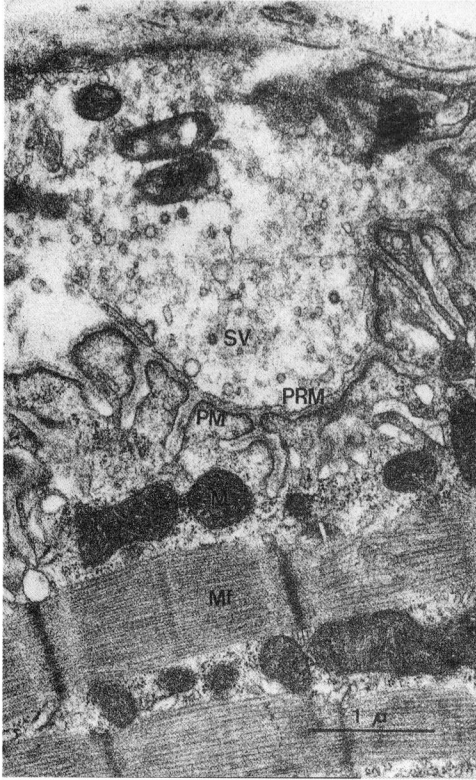

Fig. 2.5 The neuromuscular junction, demonstrating the motor nerve containing mitochondria (M) and synaptic vesicles (SV), the presynaptic membrane (PRM), the synaptic cleft and the postsynaptic membrane (PM). The muscle fibres (Mf) lie beneath the postsynaptic membrane.

ACh by producing a microcurrent, an effect blocked by tubocurare (Fig. 2.7).[17–19]

From the surface of the membrane the pentamer appears as a ring-like structure 6.5 nm diameter with a central pore of 2.5 nm. Each unit projects into the extracellular space for 5.5–6.5 nm and penetrates through the membrane as a cylindrical structure, extending 1.5–2.0 nm into the cytoplasm of the muscle. From its surface appearance it has been likened to a doughnut. Because of the repetition of two α subunits in the group of five subunits, the structure is asymmetrical, thus the α_1 unit has a β and γ (or ε) unit on each side, whilst the α_2 unit has a δ and β unit adjacent to it. This asymmetrical structure causes each AChR to have a different affinity for ACh and for non-depolarizing relaxant drugs and a slightly different response time.[20,21]

In the transmembrane plane the interior of the cylinder formed by the five subunits has a narrow isthmus where it penetrates the membrane and the different positions of the two α AChR sites are revealed (Fig. 2.8). The more rapid AChR binding site demonstrates an almost 100-fold

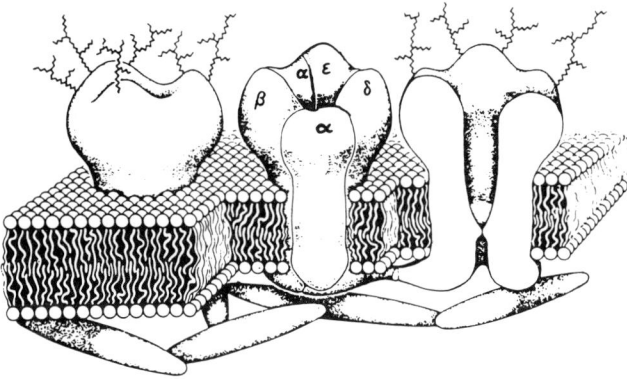

Fig. 2.6 The pentameric structure of the cholinoceptor. In the adult human the γ subunit is replaced by an ε.

difference in affinity for curare than the slower site. It is suggested that the slower site may initiate closing of the ionophore. The portion of the channel between the narrow isthmus and the extracellular collar of the pentamer is referred to as the vestibule. It is believed that the isthmus serves as the ion gate that prevents the ingress of Na^+ when the channel is closed. Activation of the AChR sites simultaneously on both α subunits will produce dilation of the isthmus, either by a twisting of the pentamer subsequent to a shortening of the α units (like a Chinese puzzle) or else by an opening of the units like the opening of the petals when a flower blooms (Fig. 2.9). The dilation of the isthmus causes the opening of the ion gate and an increase in Na^+ conductivity.

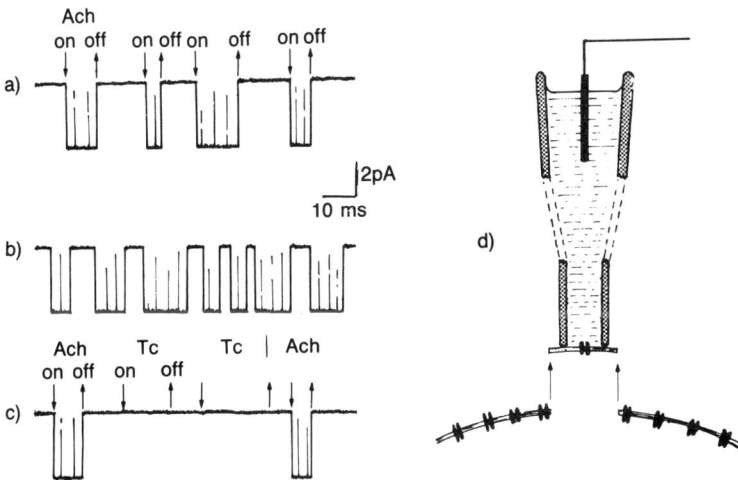

Fig. 2.7 Diagrammatic representation of (a) patch-clamp response of one cholinoceptor to acetylcholine (ACh) with a picoamp current when the channel opens – an effect blocked (c) by tubocurare (Tc). (d) Illustrates the technique by which one cholinergic receptor is sucked onto the end of a micropipette and removed from the postsynaptic membrane for study.

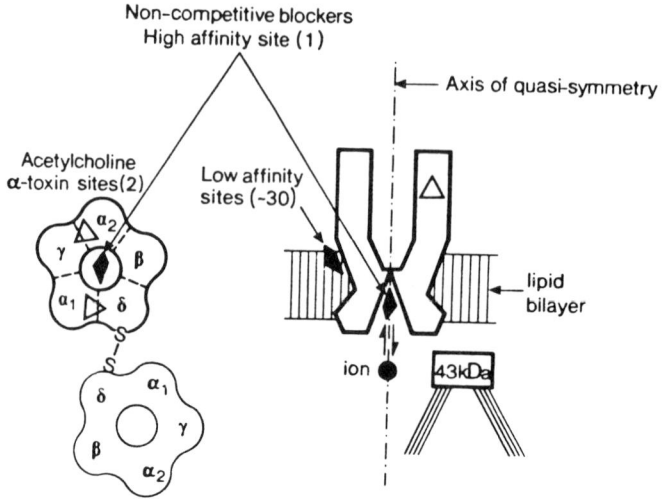

Fig. 2.8 Diagram of axial section of a cholinoceptor, demonstrating the narrow isthmus and the two α binding sites, each with a different affinity due to asymmetry of the pentamer. A high affinity channel blocking site is also indicated (1). From Galzi *et al. Ann Rev Pharmacol* 1991; **31**: 37–72.

The amino acid sequence of the helix that makes up the α subunits demonstrates four hydrophobic zones which represent the areas where the helix repeatedly penetrates the membrane. These are known as M_1–M_4. The ACh recognition zone lies at the junction of the M_2 domain with the extramembranous zone between the 30 amino acids forming the disulphide loop in the region of amino acid 172–201 on the α unit. This sequence links two sulphide bonds of cysteine molecules each with their carboxy terminal residue facing the exterior. This hairpin loop in the helix is essential for

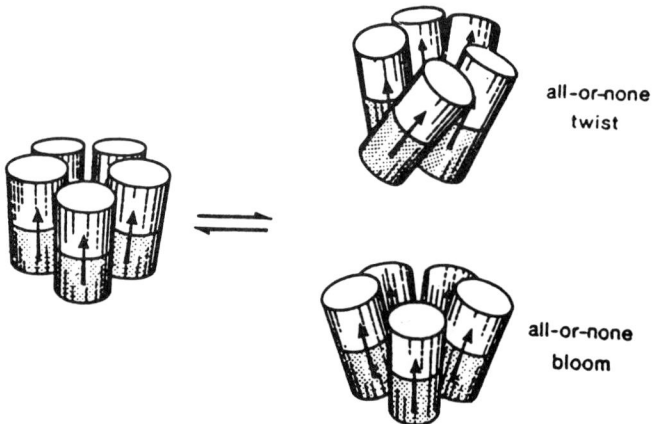

Fig. 2.9 Activation of the two acetylcholine receptors causes the five subunits to rotate, resulting in either a Chinese puzzle effect opening the central pore, or a blooming flower effect. From Galzi *et al. Ann Rev Pharmacol* 1991; **31**: 37–72.

ACh activation, which causes the ion control gate to open and Na^+ conductance to be enhanced. It is probable that residues contributed by the γ and δ subunits also form an essential part of the receptor. It has been demonstrated that chimeras of these receptors with different contributions from neighbouring subunits markedly affect their affinity for curare.[21] Activation of the recognition site on one α subunit produces cooperative facilitation of activation of the second recognition on the other α subunit.

The mammalian ACh receptor is very similar to that of *Torpedo marmorata* except that the γ unit is replaced, when the fetal structure is lost, by an ε subunit, which has a 60% similarity in amino acid sequencing. This change decreases the sensitivity of the receptor to ACh and so reduces the duration of opening of the ion channels. By means of patch-clamp techniques the opening of a single ion channel can be demonstrated to be associated with the generation of about 3–4 pA and 0.5 μV depolarization of the membrane. The mean adult channel open time to produce this minute current is of the order of 10 ms. In fetal or in the extrajunctional receptors of denervated muscle where γ subunits are found, the mean open time of the channel is up to 100 ms. However, the duration of the mean channel open time and the current produced also depends upon the resting membrane potential.[22]

The pentamer has a life cycle of about 4–6 days. There is a constant turnover and replacement of receptors in healthy innervated muscle. Following denervation and trauma the focal congregation of receptors on the postsynaptic membrane is reduced and extrajunctional receptors appear on the muscle membrane. These have the fetal structure and are short-lived (up to 2 days). The trophic influence producing the high density of normal receptors on the postjunctional membrane is believed to be calcitonin gene-related peptide, which has been demonstrated within ACh vesicles and is presumably released by normal activity[23] and a neuronally produced trophin which binds to muscle glycoprotein.

Following motor nerve denervation and as a result of loss of the trophic influence of the active motor nerve, degenerative changes appear in the postsynaptic anatomy and the normal secondary crest pattern becomes disturbed. Non-focal receptors appear on the surface of the muscle in a haphazard fashion. These extrajunctional nicotinic receptors[24] resemble fetal receptors in both composition and distribution, appearing first as clusters and then spreading more or less evenly over the membrane of the denervated muscle. The turnover rate of these extrajunctional receptors is much more rapid than that of the junctional receptors. The extrajunctional receptors have an increased sensitivity to ACh and have a longer mean open time in response to transmitter stimulation.[17] This is probably the result of the predominance of γ subunits in their structure, rather than the normal adult junctional ε. In some animals tubocurare can be demonstrated to act as an agonist on these receptors, causing membrane depolarization.[25] Agonist drugs such as suxamethonium produce prolonged channel open times, promoting the high levels of K^+ leakage which have been found to be associated with denervation injuries.[26]

In myasthenia gravis the antibodies to receptor protein cause degenerative changes in the postsynaptic membrane and a decrease in receptor population. Various antibodies have been demonstrated, including those associated with failure of one or other α subunit receptor. Myasthenia gravis is not associated with the development of extrajunctional receptors.

Up-regulation of receptors has been studied in animals in response to prolonged partial paralysis. An increase in receptor density has been demonstrated in animals after prolonged paralysis, although this effect is apparently not obvious in the all-important neuromuscular junctions in the diaphragm. It is possible that this effect may occur in patients after long-term artificial ventilation and following massive injuries.

References

1. Dale HH. The actions of certain esters and ethers of choline and their relation to muscarine. *J Pharmacol Exp Ther* 1914; **6:** 147–190
2. Waser PG & Luthi U. Autoradiographische lokalization von c-calabessen. Curarin I und c-decamethonium in der motarischen end platte. *Arch Pharmacodyn Ther* 1957; **112:** 272–296
3. Waser PG. Receptor localisation by autoradiographic techniques. *Ann NY Acad Sci* 1967; **144:** 737–755
4. Ceccarelli B & Clementi F. Neurotoxins acting at postsynaptic sites. In: *Neurotoxin Tools in Neurobiology*, vol. 3. Ceccarelli B & Clementi F (eds) New York: Raven Press (1979) pp. 141–152
5. Langley JN. On nerve endings and on special excitable substances in cells (Croonian lecture). *Proc R Soc (ser B)* 1906; **78:** 170–194
6. Langley JN. On the contraction of muscle, chiefly in relation to the presence of 'receptive' substances. *J Physiol* 1907; **36:** 347–384
7. Koelle GB. A proposed dual role of acetylcholine: its functions at the pre and post-synaptic sites. *Nature* 1961; **190:** 208–211
8. Hubbard JI, Wilson DF & Miyamoto M. Reduction of transmitter release by *d*-tubocurare. *Nature* 1969; **22:** 531
9. Hubbard JI, Sohmidt RF & Yokota T. The effect of acetylcholine upon mammalian motor nerve terminals. *J Physiol* 1965; **181:** 810–829.
10. Bowman WC & Webb SN. Tetanic fade during partial transmission failure produced by non-depolarizing neuromuscular blocking drugs in the cat. *Clin Exp Pharmacol Physiol* 1974; **3:** 545–555
11. Bowman WC. Pre and postjunctional cholinoreceptors at the neuromuscular junction. *Anesth Analg* 1980; **59:** 935–943
12. Riker WF. Prejunctional effects of neuromuscular blocking and facilitating drugs. In: *Muscle Relaxants*, Katz RL (ed.) Holland: Elsevier (1975) pp. 59–102
13. Standaert FG & Adams JE. The actions of succinylcholine on mammalian nerve terminals. *J Pharmacol Exp Ther* 1965; **149:** 113–123
14. Schwartz RD & Kellar KJ. *In vivo* regulation of ^{3}H acetylcholine recognition sites by nicotinic drugs. *J Neurochem* 1985; 427–433
15. Heinemann S, Boulter J & Deneris E. The brain nicotinic acetylcholine receptor gene family. *Prog Brain Res* 1990; **86:** 195–203
16. Silinsky EM. The biophysical pharmacology of calcium dependent acetylcholine secretion. *Pharmacol Rev* 1985; **37:** 81–132
17. Neher E & Sackman B. Single channel currents recorded from membrane of denervated frog muscle fibres. *Nature* 1976; **260:** 779–802
18. Colquhoun D & Sheridan RE. The effects of tubocurarine competition on kinetics of agonist action on the nicotinic receptor. *Br J Pharmacol* 1982; **75:** 77–86
19. Colquhoun D & Sheridan RE. The modes of action of gallamine. *Proc R Soc (Lond)* 1981; **211:** 181–203

20. Neubig RR & Cohen JB. Equilibrium binding of [H^3] tubocurarine and [H^3] acetylcholine by Torpedo postsynaptic membranes: stoichemistry and ligand interactions. *Biochemistry* 1979; **18:** 5464–5475

21. Sine S. Molecular dissection of subunit interfaces in the acetylcholine receptor. Identification of residues that determine curare selectivity. *Proc Nat Acad Sci* 1993; **90:** 9436–9440

22. Colquhoun D & Sackman B. Fluctuations in the microsecond time range of the current through single acetylcholine receptor ion channels. *Nature* 1981; **294:** 464–466

23. Sakaguchi M, Inaishim Y, Kashara K & Kuno H. Release of calcitonin gene related peptide from nerve terminals in rat skeletal muscle. *J Physiol* 1991; **434:** 257–270

24. Fambrough DM. The control of acetylcholine receptors in skeletal muscle. *Physiol Rev* 1979; **59:** 165–227

25. Takeda K & Trautman A. A patch clamp study of the partial agonist action of tubocurarine on rat myotubes. *J Physiol* 1984; **349:** 353–374

26. Gronert GA, Lambert EH & Theye RA. The response of denervated muscle to succinylcholine. *Anesthesiology* 1973; **53:** 13–17

3

Neuromuscular transmission

It was only in the late 1950s that it was finally accepted that chemical mediation was involved in the transmission of the nerve action potential to the muscle fibre to bring about muscle contraction. Up to that time Eccles and others had argued that acetylcholine (ACh) release was incidental to an essentially physical process of electrical signal propagation from nerve to muscle.

It is now completely accepted that motor nerve activation produces a release of ACh at the nerve terminal and that this excites the membrane of the muscle. If this excitation reaches a critical level it will trigger a propagated action potential, resulting in muscle contraction.

The nerve action potential is carried from one node of Ranvier to the next by saltatory conduction. It is associated with activation of sodium and potassium channels. Once the wave of excitation reaches the nerve ending inside the synaptic cleft – the prejunctional membrane – voltage gated calcium channels are activated, resulting in an influx of the Ca^{2+} ions necessary to trigger the release of ACh. The sodium and potassium channels of the nerve axon are cation-specific and blocked by different drugs, i.e. tetrodotoxin blocks Na^+ channels and aminopyridine blocks the K^+ channels. The calcium channels are associated with the active zones of the presynaptic membrane.

Released ACh diffuses across the synaptic cleft and activates the postsynaptic nicotinic receptors embodied in the postsynaptic membrane on the shoulders of the secondary clefts. These receptors control the postsynaptic ion channel. These channels are not specific for either sodium or potassium. However, in the resting state the narrowness of the isthmus restricts the passage of larger hydrated Na^+ ion. It is the selective ability of K^+ to traverse the membrane along its electrochemical gradient, in the resting state, that produces the resting membrane potential. Once an ion channel is open and Na^+ as well as K^+ can pass through the activated receptor channel, a local fall in membrane potential will occur associated with a picoamp (2–3 pA) current. The total current produced will be proportional to the number of channels opened simultaneously. Thus, the ease with which membrane depolarization occurs depends upon the number of receptors activated simultaneously and the resting membrane potential. A reduction of the resting membrane potential from −90 to −55.0 mV is critical if a propagated action potential is to occur and muscle contraction is to be produced.[1] The critical level of depolarization required to produce a propagated action potential is probably dependent upon many factors, including the level of the resting membrane potential, the composition of the environment surrounding the receptors and the animal species. The ease with which the propagated action potential produces muscle contraction may be affected by external Ca^{2+} concentration, muscle temperature, drugs and, in certain animals, the activity of perijunctional receptors. These double-gated channels respond to a combination of chemical transmitters and changes in electrical potential in the adjacent membrane.

The membrane potential

The difference between the inside of the resting muscle membrane and the extracellular or synaptic cleft surface at rest is about −90 mV. This is the resting membrane potential. The excitability of the neuromuscular junction and its response to ACh depends upon the magnitude of this transmembrane potential. The membrane potential is a consequence of the apparent selective permeability of the membrane at rest and is consequent upon the unequal distribution of ions on the two sides of this apparently semipermeable membrane. The Nearnst equation describes the electromotive force (emf) generated across a semipermeable membrane in terms of the concentrations of the most permeable ion: in the resting state, this ion is potassium. As a result the Nearnst equation can be represented as:

$$\text{emf} = \frac{RT}{F} \log_e \frac{[K^o]}{[K^i]}$$

where R is the universal gas constant, T is the absolute temperature, F is the Faraday constant, $[K^o]$ is the concentration of potassium in extracellular water and $[K^i]$ that in the intracellular fluid. This expression ignores the small contribution of anions and the minor effect of Na^+. The Hodgkin–Katz formula, which takes these into account, provides an even more accurate forecast of the transmembrane potential. However, the effect of these additional ions is small and for practical purposes in humans it is the ratio of extracellular to intracellular K^+ concentration that determines the resting membrane potential.

The resting transmembrane potential can be envisaged as the result of K^+ ions moving along their concentration gradient from the inside of the cell, where they are 50 times more concentrated, towards the extracellular fluid (ECF). As the membrane is permeable to K^+, this movement will continue until it produces an excess of positively charged ions on the outside of the membrane. When the electrostatic potential is sufficient to prevent the further egress of the positively charged K^+ from the cell, equilibrium will be produced. At this point the potential across the membrane will be −90 mV. If the concentration of K^+ in the ECF is raised or the intracellular K^+ decreased, then equilibrium will be reached at a lower potential.

It is evident, therefore, that the resting membrane potential depends upon the ratio of the $[K^i]/[K^o]$, not upon any absolute value. In normal circumstances this ratio is approximately $50/1$ ($[K^i] = 150$ mmol, $[K^o] = 5$ mmol). If the ratio is increased then the resting membrane potential is increased and it becomes more difficult to produce critical depolarization. As a result, it appears resistant to ACh and sensitive to non-depolarizing drugs. Conversely, if the ratio is decreased then there will be an apparent resistance to non-depolarizing drugs. With the normal values for potassium inside and outside the cell and a normal total body potassium, small shifts of 1 or 2 mmol make little impact on the ratio and upon the resting membrane potential. However, in circumstances of total body potassium depletion, such as prolonged diarrhoea or long-term use of a loop diuretic, then the same 1–2 mmol shift in potassium will have an exaggerated effect.[2] This might explain some of the cases of cardiac arrest that have followed the use of suxamethonium in patients with chronic potassium loss from renal disease. The circumstances in which the ratio of intracellular to extracellular potassium is disturbed are relatively rare; they include familial periodic paralysis, mucus-secreting tumours of the bowel, steroid overdose, the administration of glucose and insulin, acute alkalaemia and following anoxia. In most circumstances of chronic potassium loss the reduction in K^+ is distributed between the intracellular and extracellular spaces to maintain a normal ratio and hence a normal response to muscle relaxants. In the presence of total body K^+ depletion relatively small shifts of potassium may produce an exaggerated change in transmembrane potential. This effect usually produces cardiac arrhythmias and even cardiac arrest; it will not, however, affect sensitivity to muscle relaxant drugs.

The rapid inflow of Na^+ ions that occurs when the receptors are activated is associated with a voltage change which will trigger an action potential when it exceeds the critical threshold. This is followed by a late, slower inflow of K^+ ions to restore the electrostatic gradient prior to the outflow of excess Na^+ (Fig. 3.1).

Activation of the cholinoceptor

The postsynaptic ACh receptor (cholinoceptor) is a large structure surrounding the central ion channel. Only a small part of this structure responds to ACh. The ACh receptor recognition sites are principally situated on the two α subunits, where they involve a sequence of some 30 amino acids. Both recognition sites need to be activated simultaneously to produce the increase in Na^+ conductance necessary for local depolarization of the membrane. The two units have different affinities and response times, although activation of one receptor co-operatively influences the ACh occupancy of the other receptor. The low-affinity receptor reacts more slowly to ACh and is believed to play an important role in closing the ion gate.[3] The receptor sites also have very different affinities for antagonist drugs.[4,5] There is good evidence that non-depolarizing drugs combine reversibility with multiple sites with affinities that differ as much as 100-fold, depending upon the chimera of the adjacent subunit

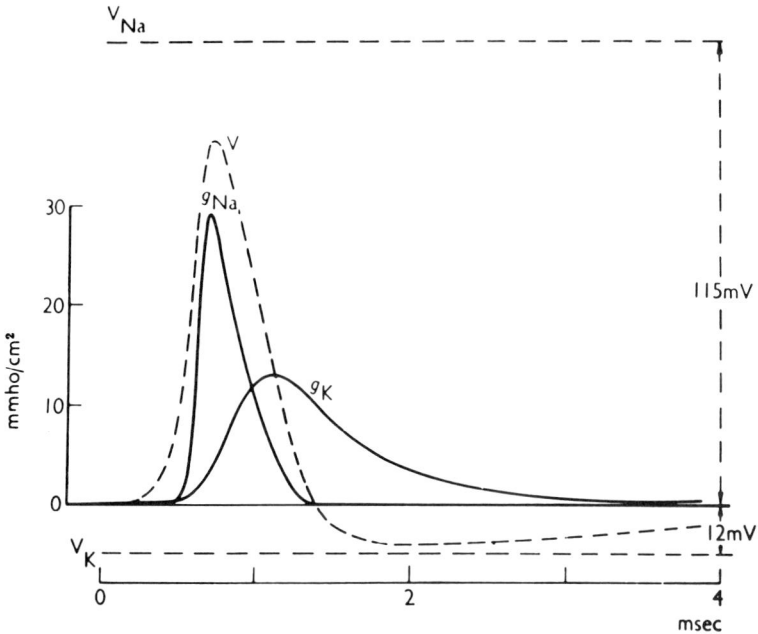

Fig. 3.1 The relationship between Na^+, K^+ flux and the end-plate potential change during end-plate activation. From Hodgkin and Harrowitz.

incorporated in the α receptor.[6] Occupancy of either one of two ACh recognition sites will prevent ACh from activating the receptors. The affinity of most antagonists for an ACh recognition site is many times that of ACh. As a result, the competition between ACh and an antagonist drug for receptor occupancy is always biased in favour of the neuro-muscular blocking drug.

References

1. Jenerick HP & Gerrard RW. Membrane potential and threshold of single muscle fibre. *J Cell Comp Physiol* 1953; **42:** 79–83
2. Feldman SA. Effects of changes in electrolytes, hydration and pH upon reactions to muscle relaxants. *Br J Anaesth* 1963; **35:** 546–549
3. Jackson MB. Performance of a synaptic receptor: kinetics and energetics of the acetylcholine receptor. *Proc Nat Acad Sci USA* 1989; **86:** 2199–2203
4. Sine SM & Taylor P. Relationship between reversible antagonist occupancy and the functional capacity of the acetylcholine receptor. *J Biol Chem* 1981; **256:** 6692–6699
5. Pedersen SE & Cohen JB. *d*-tubocurarine binding sites are located at alpha-gamma and alpha-delta subunit interfaces of the nicotinic acetylcholine receptor. *Proc Natl Acad Sci* 1990; **87:** 2785–2789
6. Sine SM. Molecular dissection of subunit interfaces in the acetylcholine receptor. Identification of residues that determine curare selectivity. *Proc Natl Acad Sci* 1993; **90:** 9436–9440
7. Hodgkin AL & Harrowitz P. The influence of potassium and chloride ions on the membrane potential of single muscle fibres. *J Physiol (Lond)* **148:** 127–141

4

Acetylcholine formation and metabolism

Acetylcholine (ACh) is formed principally in the axoplasm of the motor nerve terminal by the acetylation of choline. A small amount may be formed in the neuron and pass by axonal transport to the region of the motor nerve ending. Similarly, a small amount of ACh appears to be synthesized by the Schwann cells and to be released from within the myelin sheath in the end-plate region.

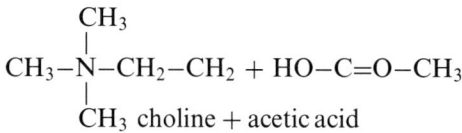

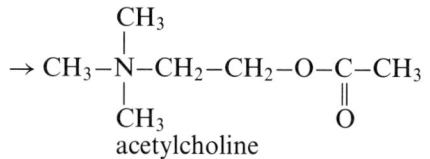

$$CH_3-\underset{\underset{CH_3}{|}}{\overset{\overset{CH_3}{|}}{N}}-CH_2-CH_2 + HO-C=O-CH_3$$
choline + acetic acid

$$\rightarrow CH_3-\underset{\underset{CH_3}{|}}{\overset{\overset{CH_3}{|}}{N}}-CH_2-CH_2-O-\underset{\underset{O}{\|}}{C}-CH_3$$
acetylcholine

Acetylcholine is synthesized by the large mitochondria in the axoplasm from choline and acetylated by coenzyme A (choline-o-acetyltransferase). The choline substrate is not synthesized at the nerve terminal but comes from choline in the plasma; about 50% of this is the choline that is recycled as the result of hydrolysis of ACh by acetylcholinesterase in the synaptic cleft.[1] Choline requires active transport across the motor nerve membrane in order to enter the axoplasm. This is achieved by a sodium-dependent high-affinity pump mechanism, not found outside the nervous system, with a rapid dissociation constant.[2] Blockade of this carrier process by drugs such as hemicholinium causes a rundown of ACh which *in vivo* causes a myasthenic-like syndrome of muscle weakness which is particularly obvious on exercise. The closely related triethyl compound, triethylcholine, has similar properties which have been attributed to its action as a 'false' choline base which is acetylated in the axoplasm to produce the acetyl derivative which acts as a false transmitter substance.[3] Although coenzyme A (choline-o-acetyltransferase) can be demonstrated in the synaptic vesicles, it is believed that the major part of the synthesis of ACh occurs in mitochondria in the axoplasm.[4,5]

Acetylcholine is first produced in solution in the axoplasm and has to be 'packaged' into vesicles before it can be released as a transmitter in a sufficiently concentrated form to produce neurotransmission. The synaptic vesicles are synthesized in the neuronal body and pass by axonal micro-tubular transport to the nerve terminal.[6] The membrane surrounding the vesicles is a complex structure and is important in modifying ACh storage and release. Although there appears to be a constant small leakage of free non-vesicular ACh from the axoplasm, which increases especially upon motor nerve stimulation, the bulk of the evidence suggests that it does not play a major role in neuromuscular transmission.[7]

ACh is packaged into vesicles against a 10-fold concentration gradient utilizing an adenosine triphosphatase (ATPase)-dependent mechanism to exchange intravesicular protons for cytoplasmic ACh.[8] The vesicles involved in this process, at slow rates of motor stimulation, are principally those that have recently emptied their contents into the synaptic cleft. This constitutes the vesicular recycling process.[9] Serial autoradiographic studies have demonstrated these empty vesicles refilling with ACh.[10] The recharging of the vesicles must require energy and a pump mechanism. This indicates the complexity of the membranes of the vesicles. It is now appreciated that these structures incorporate several discrete receptor mechanisms which are of some consequence in understanding the action of toxins on neuromuscular transmission. The process of concentrating ACh in the vesicles can be interfered with by various drugs, of which vesamicol has been extensively studied. This drug, like the similar-acting tetraphenylboron, is believed not to affect the ACh–ATPase transport system directly but to produce its effect on the vesicle itself. It produces inhibition of the ACh-concentrating mechanism and results in a slow run-down of neuromuscular transmission and eventually produces neuro-muscular block.[11–13]

ACh exists in the axoplasm and within the synaptic vesicles. However, it has been demonstrated that not all the synaptic vesicles are in an immediately releasable form.[14] Studies during slow rates of stimulation suggest that the rapid turnover of ACh occurs from the small, readily releasable store of synaptic vesicles that are constantly recycled, leaving a much larger number of synaptic vesicles in reserve. The reserve vesicles, which are morphologically indistinguishable from the readily releasable vesicle forms, are a large reserve store which is mobilized when tetanic rates of stimulation are used. Estimates suggest that for every releasable vesicle there are 100–200 reserve vesicles.[15] It is now appreciated that the reserve vesicles require Ca^{2+} ions to free them from a phosphoprotein restraint before they can take part in neuromuscular transmission and that they function as an 'in-depth' reserve called upon at motor nerve stimulation over 0.5 Hz and in times of tetanic rates of motor nerve activity (Fig. 4.1). Failure of this mobilization is believed to be the cause of tetanic fade.

It is postulated that, following prolonged, high-frequency motor nerve stimulation, ACh feedback activates presynaptic nicotinic receptors, facilitating an influx of Ca^{2+} into the axoplasm (see Chapter 10). The Ca^{2+}

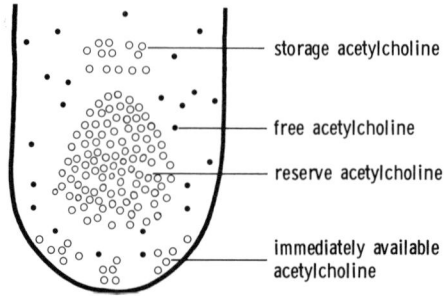

Fig. 4.1 Schematic representation of the distribution of acetylcholine in the resting motor nerve. The reserve and storage acetylcholine vesicles constitute over 90% of the acetylcholine in the nerve.

ions have two principal effects; they cause fusion of a component of the synaptic vesicles, syntaxin, with α latrotoxin receptors in the active zone of the presynaptic nerve membrane.[16,17] This causes exocytosis of the vesicle and discharge of the ACh content into the synaptic cleft. The active zones of the presynaptic nerve terminal appear as the holes in a rectangular lattice covering the membrane. With high-power resolution it is found that they consist of four rows of pairs of particles which are believed to be involved in the Ca^{2+} channels.[18] The migration of the vesicles to the receptive active zone of the presynaptic membrane involves activation of the glycoproteins synaptophysin and synaptotagmin on the surface of the vesicle. The second action caused by the influx of Ca^{2+} is to mobilize reserve vesicles by an action on synapsin I, a complex phosphoprotein which forms part of the vesicle. The Ca^{2+} causes phosphorylation of ATPase which activates the separation of the serine residue in the tail of synapsin I from microtubular filaments in the axoplasm, liberating the vesicle from its enveloping restraints. This mechanism involves activation of calmodulin by Ca^{2+} and a subsequent effect on ATPase[19,20] (Fig. 4.2).

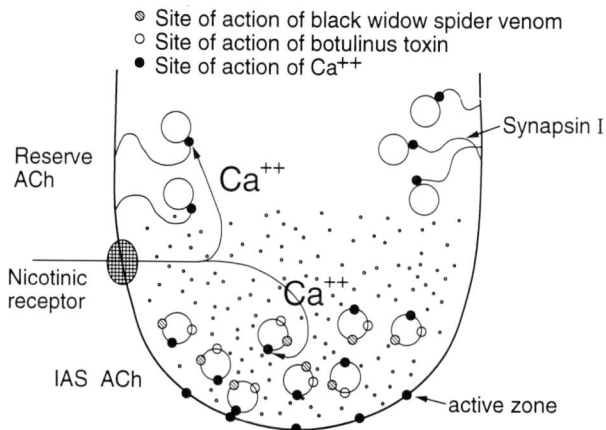

Fig. 4.2 This diagram (after Bowman[6]) indicates the two important roles of Ca^{2+} in mobilizing reserve acetylcholine (ACh) and releasing ACh into the synaptic cleft. The prejunctional nicotinic receptors (n_{mob}) are primarily involved in the first activity. IAS = immediately available ACh

As a result of this exquisitely balanced feedback mechanism, the supply of ACh can be increased to meet the needs of increased motor nerve activity in exercise. As the number of releasable vesicles increases in the presynaptic nerve terminal, the number of ACh vesicles randomly liberated in response to neural stimulation will increase to meet the period of peak demand. Once motor nerve activity ceases there is a short period before the proportion of vesicles in the releasable state is reduced once again to the resting level and the ratio of reserve vesicles to active vesicles is re-established. During this time a further stimulation of the motor nerve releases more ACh than when the status quo has been re-established. This is the basis of the phenomenon of post-tetanic potentiation (Fig. 4.3).

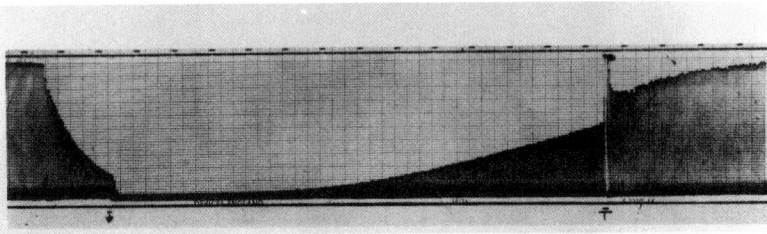

Fig. 4.3 Tetanic stimulus (T) of 100 Hz causes decurarization by increased acetylcholine mobilization and release. This phenomenon is seen if the plasma level of the drug is low.

(This should be distinguished from the increase in twitch response due to post-tetanic enhancement – a purely muscle effect.) Repeated bursts of tetanic stimulation may increase the rate of ACh production and act rather like small localized injections of ACh in hastening the recovery of neuromuscular transmission following neuromuscular block[21,22] (Fig. 4.4).

The function of the synaptic vesicle is important in understanding how various animal and plant toxins effect their action. Botulinus toxin reacts with a specific receptor (synaptobrevin) on the surface of the vesicle to stabilize the structure, preventing it from taking part in neuromuscular transmission. The resulting rundown in available ACh produces muscle weakness and paralysis.[16] Black widow spider venom (α latrotoxin) causes a massive release of ACh as a result of its action at a specific latrotoxin receptor on the presynaptic membrane. Once the stores of ACh vesicles have been exhausted, the toxin prevents refilling and docking with syntaxin in the active zone of the presynaptic membrane.[21] The venom causes muscle spasm and tachycardia, followed by muscle weakness and respiratory failure. Other less studied putative receptors on the vesicles have been suggested but their role in ACh formation and release has been less well-studied. Various toxins act on the presynaptic ACh mechanism, whilst others such as conotoxin and bungarotoxin act at postsynaptic sites (Fig. 4.5).

(a)

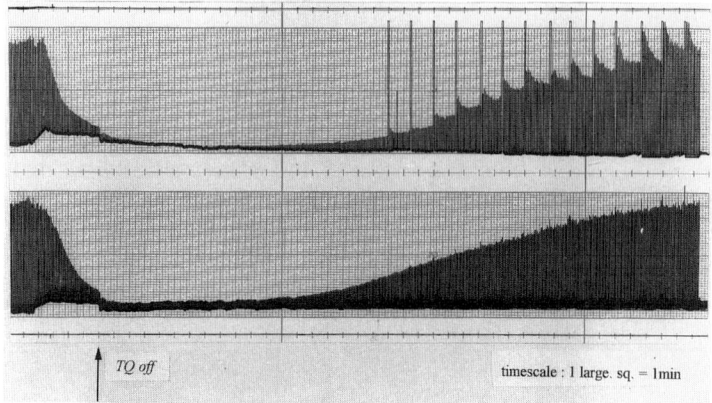

TQ off

timescale : 1 large. sq. = 1min

VECURONIUM 0.3mg

(b)

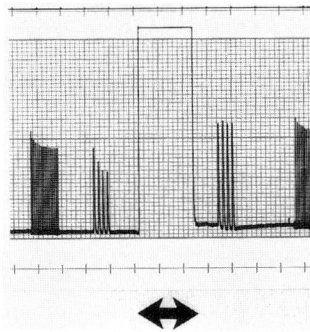

VOLUNTARY TETANUS

Fig. 4.4 (a) Repeated tetanic stimulation (voluntary muscle contraction) causes an increased rate of reversal of neuromuscular block. From Gopinath et al.[22] with permission. (b) Tetanic contraction causes reversal of train-of-four fade.

Presynaptic action of acetylcholine (see Chapter 10)

In addition to its action on the postsynaptic receptor mechanism, ACh also acts as a neurotransmitter at muscarinc receptors in autonomic ganglia, in the heart and in neural transmission in the central nervous system. It is hardly surprising therefore that it also affects presynaptic receptors on nerve terminals. It has been suggested that there are different prejunctional receptors, some affecting the feedback mechanism, n_{mob}, and others responsible for repetitive afterdischarge following motor nerve stimulation, n_{rep}. There is evidence that the presynaptic receptors exposed to very high concentrations of ACh become insensitive or actually cause a negative

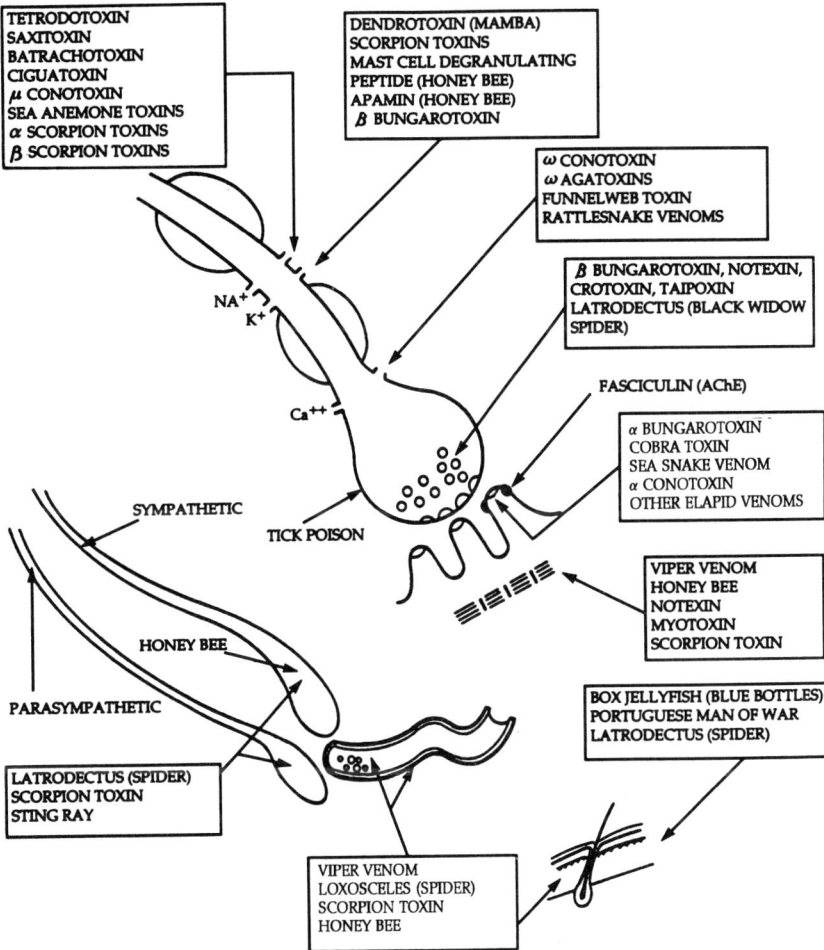

Fig. 4.5 Sites of action of animal toxins affecting the neuromuscular junction. ACht = Acetylcholinesterase. Courtesy of Dr L. Karelliedde.

feedback on ACh synthesis and mobilization. However, without identifying the receptors, all of the proposed actions have to be inferred from pharmacological responses. The other difficulty in studying these effects is the ease with which desensitization occurs. Indeed, brief stimulation followed by prolonged desensitization characterizes the response of these receptors. It seems reasonable to anticipate that the presynaptic nicotinic receptors will prove to be similar to the family of neural nicotinic receptors. The central nervous system lacks the genes to express γ or δ subunits and as a result produces a series of simpler pentamers than those at the postsynaptic membrane. It is possible that this simplified structure is responsible for the different kinetic pattern of ACh and agonist and antagonist drugs acting at this site.

Clinical importance of presynaptic feedback

Various clinical observations, such as the presence of train-of-four (TOF) fade at 2 Hz stimulation of the motor nerve and tetanic fade are taken as evidence of presynaptic block of the feedback mechanism. However, although it does not constitute proof that such a mechanism is involved, it does appear to be plausible.[23] The consistency with which TOF fade is found, especially upon recovery from non-depolarizing block suggests that all these drugs, at least in the recovery phase of their block, produce both presynaptic and postsynaptic events.

The rundown of ACh release at higher rates of stimulation is the probable explanation of the observed reduction of 50% in the onset time of rocuronium block when the rate of motor nerve stimulation was increased from 0.1 to 1.0 Hz.[24] Recent work in our laboratory on the rat phrenic nerve diaphragm has suggested an exponential increase in the rate of onset of rocuronium block as the rate of nerve stimulation was increased from 0.1 to 5 Hz. Above this rate of stimulation the relationship was virtually linear. As this effect is not observed during block by α-bungaro-toxin, it suggests that it is due to an early presynaptic block by rocuronium increasingly revealed at higher rates of stimulation.[25]

Postsynaptic action of acetylcholine

Fatt and Katz[26] recorded small end-plate potentials occurring in frog muscle fibres at rest. The miniature end-plate potentials (MEPP) they described are due to the random discharge of synaptic vesicles into the synaptic cleft. The low current recorded is generated by the opening of a limited number of Na^+ channels on the postsynaptic membrane. The size and frequency of their occurrence suggest that they represent discrete events or summation of two or three such events. It is believed that the unit of the MEPP represents the discharge of a single ACh vesicle into the synaptic cleft and suggests a uniform number of ACh molecules – between 6000 and 10000 in each vesicle. By studying the random frequency of this end-plate current and the effect of drugs on the size and frequency of the MEPPs, their effect on the ACh contents of vesicle can be assessed (Fig. 4.6).

Following motor nerve stimulation, an action potential is conducted from one node of Ranvier to the next by saltatory conduction until it reaches the preterminal region where the myelin sheath terminates. At the terminal region the density of Na^+ channels found on the motor nerve is reduced and, once beyond the myelin sheath, neural activation occurs as a result of K^+ channel activity. It can be demonstrated that the inwards Na^+ activity in the nerve is associated with an outward passage of K^+ in the terminal zone. It is the opening of the K^+ channels and the outward passage of K^+ that promote the inward migration of Ca^{2+} in the nerve terminal. It is this voltage gated Ca^{2+} transport that results in the massive discharge of ACh content of the releasable vesicles into the synaptic cleft,

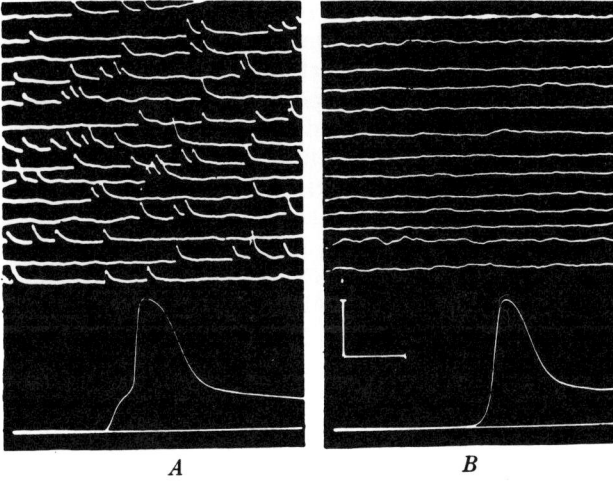

Fig. 4.6 Intracellular recording taken at the end-plate (A) and at a distance of 2 mm in a frog muscle fibre (B). The upper part, taken at low speed (47 ms) and high amplification (3.6 mV), shows the presence of miniature end-plate potentials only in the recording taken at the end-plate site. The lower part, taken at high speed (2 ms) and low amplification (50 mV), shows the response to a nerve stimulus. Note the initial slower rate of depolarization (the end-plate potential) in trace A. From Fatt and Katz,[26] with permission.

which in turn produces postsynaptic depolarization (Fig. 4.7). If the post-synaptic current produced exceeds the threshold value, a self-propagating action potential will be produced and muscle contraction will result. It has been calculated that a considerable excess of ACh is released pre-synaptically, compared to that required to produce the end-plate current and trigger an action potential.

Recent work suggests that the original figure of 300 000–400 000 molecules of ACh is too high for humans. Indeed, the excess release of ACh

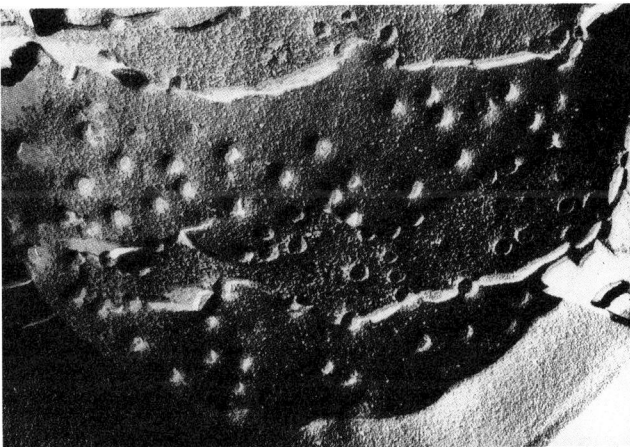

Fig. 4.7 Synaptic vesicles being released from presynaptic membrane.

appears to be greatest in lower animal species and hibernating animals and least in homothermic mammals and humans. The released ACh has to pass across the 20 nm gap of the synaptic cleft, within which lies a mesh of basement membrane filaments largely composed of mucopolysaccharide, in the interstices of which are the long-tailed molecules of acetylcholinesterase. The anatomical coincidence of the active zones of the presynaptic membrane and the crests of secondary clefts on the postsynaptic membrane, with its high density of receptors, suggests that a mechanism may exist to limit the exposure of released ACh to the acetylcholinesterase in the cleft during its passage to the ACh receptor. However, on leaving the ACh receptor, the molecules of ACh are less likely to benefit from this limitation of exposure to cholinesterase.

Metabolism of acetylcholine

ACh is rapidly hydrolysed by acetylcholinesterase in the synaptic cleft. The neurotransmitter has a half-life of 1–2 ms. The hydrolysis occurs in several steps. ACh combines with acetylcholinesterase at the quaternary nitrogen head by electrostatic forces, whilst the carbomate group on the enzyme splits off the choline. The acetylated enzyme is reconstituted by the reaction of the acetyl residue with water.

Neostigmine and related amino carbomate esters and edrophonium react with acetylcholinesterase to form stable inactive compounds that prevent the enzyme hydrolysing ACh and so prolong the half-life of the transmitter in the synaptic cleft.

Acetylcholinesterase inhibitors – anticholinesterase drugs

The two principal anticholinesterase drugs used in clinical anaesthesia are neostigmine and edrophonium. Pyridostigmine is widely used in the treatment of myasthenia gravis but its long duration of action is unnecessary to reverse residual neuromuscular block.

Edrophonium (Tensilon; Fig. 4.8) is believed to exert its anticholinesterase activity by combining with the enzyme by means of weak electrostatic bonds. The time of onset is very rapid (<1 ms), whilst the dissociation rate, K_{off}, is less than 30 s. In *in vivo* experiments its anticholinesterase action has been estimated to decline to about 45% activity in 10 min and 15% at 20 min following a large dose (0.5 mg/kg).[27] Although one would anticipate that there would be a prolongation of the anticholinesterase effect as the dose was increased, it is found that there is only a minor effect when the dose is increased from 0.125 to 0.5 mg/kg and that, even with the largest dose, the effect has usually completely worn off after 50 min.[28]

Neostigmine (Fig. 4.8) acts as a substrate for cholinesterase. However, when the amino carbomate is hydrolysed, the carbomate forms a strong bond with the enzyme. The carbomylated enzyme is inactive and its esterase activity is inhibited. The dynamics of the process are slower than edrophonium, being about 50% complete in 65 s. Complete inhibition of

EDROPHONIUM

ACETYLCHOLINESTERASE

NEOSTIGMINE

ACETYLCHOLINESTERASE

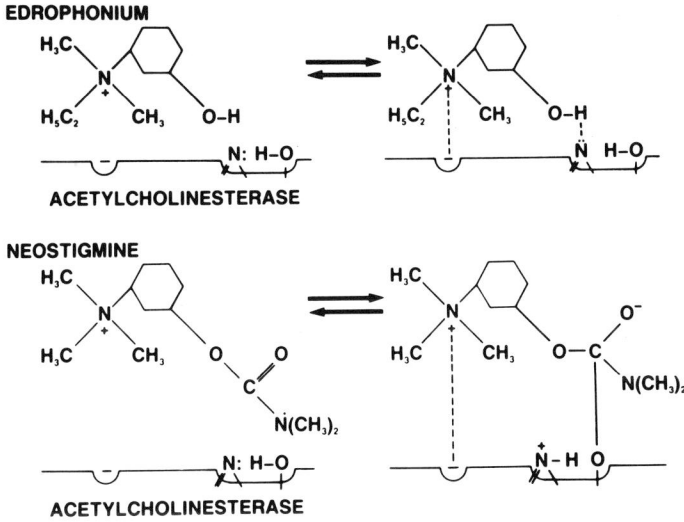

Fig. 4.8 Proposed mechanism of inhibition of acetylcholinesterase by edrophonium and neostigmine.

the enzyme may take 8–10 min. The plasma half-life of neostigmine is very similar to that of an equipotent dose of edrophonium, although its anti-cholinesterase action is considerably longer. It is possible that this is a reflection of the slow dissociation constant of the carbomate–enzyme bond. The clinical effect of pyridostimine is in the order of 6–8 h, although the *in vitro* cholinesterase effect is of a similar duration to neostigmine. No explanation of this pharmacokinetic paradox has been suggested.

Hobbiger[29] illustrated the importance of the anticholinesterase effect in reversing residual curare block by demonstrating the much reduced effect of the muscle relaxant drugs if the acetylcholinesterase had previously been inhibited. Recent work has clearly demonstrated an additional alternative site of action of neostigmine. Braga *et al.*[30] found that, even after complete inhibition of acetylcholinesterase by DFP there could be up to 37% of the reversal action by neostigmine, compared with its effect before inhibition by DFP.

The possibility of a postsynaptic action of neostigmine has also been suggested by the finding that it will produce an end-plate current in isolated receptors and that the muscle contraction produced by close intra-arterial injection of the drug is abolished after the pretreatment with α-bungarotoxin. However, it is the demonstration of significant presynaptic effects of both neostigmine and edrophonium that probably accounts for the actions of these drugs after DFP inhibition of anticholinesterase. The repetitive firing seen after motor nerve stimulation in the presence of edrophonium and neostigmine suggests that such a mechanism exists. Blaber[31] has demonstrated an increase in ACh output presynaptically in the presence of edrophonium. Although this could possibly be explained as a feedback mechanism caused by the prolonged half-life of released ACh, this finding, together with other evidence of presynaptic activity of these drugs and the inability to explain other observed occurrences on the basis of the inhibition of cholinesterase alone, makes the suggestion of a major presynaptic action of the anticholinesterases an attractive hypothesis.

Clinical paradoxes

The long duration of the acetylcholinesterase inhibition produced *in vitro* by neostigmine and the long half-life of both neostigmine and higher doses of edrophonium (Fig. 4.9) would be expected to produce profound, prolonged inhibition of ACh hydrolysis with both drugs.

It would be expected that following a large dose of neostigmine (0.05 mg/kg), any attempt to produce a non-depolarizing block by a subsequent administration of drug would be frustrated or only partially successful. In practice, 5 min after administration of this dose of neostigmine it is possible to produce 100% block using a $2 \times ED_{95}$ dose of vecuronium. It is even more surprising to find that the block is produced at the same rate as with the original administration.[32]

As a result, it would also be anticipated that, on the basis of the competition theory, residual neuromuscular block by a non-depolarizing drug should always be fully reversible by an adequate dose of anticholinesterase. Clearly this is not the case and this is one of the arguments in favour of a biophase binding reservoir (see Chapter 7).

It is a fairly consistent finding that, as expected from the chemistry involved, edrophonium has a more rapid reversal effect on neuromuscular block compared with neostigmine. However, in deeper degrees of block this initial effect usually wanes in 5–10 min. Neostigmine is invariably found to provide better long-term reversal from deeper degrees of neuromuscular block than edrophonium.[28]

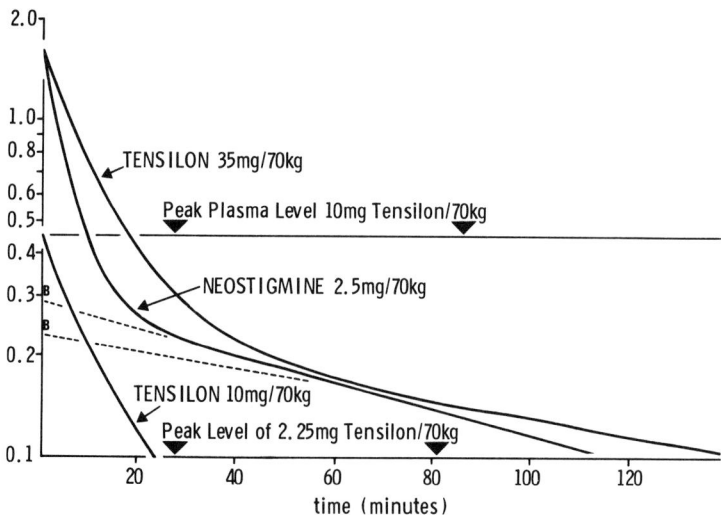

Fig. 4.9 Plasma concentrations of edrophonium (Tensilon) and neostigmine, demonstrating prolonged equal plasma concentrations of neostigmine and high-dose edrophonium. After Kopman.[28]

References

1. Collier B & Mackintosh FC. The source of choline for acetylcholine synthesis in a sympathetic ganglion. *Can J Physiol Pharmacol* 1968; **47**: 127–133

2. Yamamura HI & Snyder SH. Affinity transport of choline into synaptosomes of rat brain. *J Neurochem* 1973; **21**: 1355–1374

3. Vaca K & Pilar G. Mechanism controlling choline transport and acetylcholine synthesis in motor nerve terminals during electrical stimulation. *J Gen Physiol* 1979; **73**: 605–628.

4. Beach RL, Vaca K & Pilar G. Ionic and metabolic requirements for high affinity choline uptake and acetylcholine synthesis in nerve terminals of a neuromuscular junction. *J Neurochem* 1980; **34**: 1387–1398

5. Potter LT. (1968) Uptake of choline by nerve endings isolated from the rat cerebral cortex. In: *The Interaction of Drugs and Subcellular Components of Animal Cells* Campbell PN (ed.). London: Churchill Livingstone

6. Bowman WC. The neuromuscular junction, recent developments. *Eur J Anaesthesiol* 1985 **2**: 59–93

7. Katz B & Meiledi R. Does the motor nerve impulse evoke non-quantal transmitter release? *Proc R Soc Lond Ser B* 1981; **212**: 131–137

8. Marshall IG & Prior C. (1994) Update on the acetylcholine receptor and the neuromuscular junction. In: *Baillières Clinical Anaesthesiology*, vol. 8. Goldhill DR & Flynn PJ (eds). London: Bailliere Tindall, pp. 299–313

9. Parsons SM, Prior C & Marshall IG. Acetylcholine transport, storage and release. *Int Rev Neurobiol* 1993; **35**: 279–390

10. Waser PG, Osterwalder M & Schonenberger F. Autoradiography of C^{14} choline uptake in the endplates of skeletal muscle. *Naunyn Schmiedebergs Arch Pharmacol* 1978; **302**: 173–179

11. Anderson DC, King SC & Parsons SM. Inhibition of [H^3] acetylcholine active transport by tetraphenylborate and other ions. *Mol Pharmacol* 1983; **24**: 55–59

12. Marshall IG & Parsons SM. The vesicular acetylcholine transport system. *Trends Neurosci* 1987; **10**: 174–177

13. Marshall IG & Parsons SM. The effects of tetraphenylboron on neuromuscular transmission in the frog. *Br J Pharmacol* 1975; **54**: 333–338

14. Birks RI & MacIntosh FC. Acetylcholine metabolism of a sympathetic ganglion. *Can J Biochem Physiol* 1961; **39**: 787–827.

15. Glavinovic MI & Narahashi T. Depression, recovery and facilitation of neuromuscular transmission during prolonged tetanic stimulation. *Neurosciences* 1988; **25**: 271–281

16. Frontali N, Ceccerelli B, Gario A *et al*. Purification from black widow spider venom of a protein causing depletion of synaptic vesicles at neuromuscular junctions. *J Cell Biol* 1976; **68**: 462–479

17. Petrenko AG, Perin MS, Davletov BA *et al*. Binding of synaptognium to α latrotoxin receptor implicates both in synaptic vesicles exocytosis. *Nature* 1991; **353**: 65–68

18. Fukunaga H, Engel AG, Osome M & Lambert EH. Paucity and disorganisation of presynaptic membrane active zones in Eaton–Lambert myasthenic syndrome. *Muscle Nerve* 1982; **5**: 686–697

19. de Camilli P, Bontenati F, Valtorta F & Greengard P. The synapsins. *Annu Rev Cell Biol* 1990; **6**: 3–460

20. Benfenati F, Valtarta F, Rubenstein J *et al*. Synaptic vesicles associated Ca^{2+}/calmodulin-dependent protein kinase II as a binding protein for synapsin I. *Nature* 1992; **359**: 417–420

21. Schiavo G, Benfenati F, Poulain B *et al*. Tetanus and botulinium B block neurotransmitter release by cleavage of synaptobrevin. *Nature* 1992; **359**: 832–834

22. Gopinath S, Hood JR, Ul Haq *et al*. Effect of voluntary tetanus on recovery of vecuronium in the isolated forearm. *Anaesthesia* 1993; **48**: 870–872

23. Feldman S. Second thoughts on the train of four. *Anaesthesia* 1993; **48**: 1–2

24. Feldman SA & Khaw K. The effect of variations in the dose on the action of rocuronium with observations on the effects of the rate of stimulation. *Eur J Anaesthesiol* 1995; **125:** 15–17

25. Redai I, Richards K, England A & Feldman SA. The effect of rate of stimulation on onset of neuromuscular block in rat phrenic nerve diaphragm. *ARS* Nov 1995

26. Fatt P & Katz B. Spontaneous sub threshold activity at motor nerve endings. *J Physiol* 1951; **115:** 320–370

27. Calvey TB, Williams NE, Muir KT & Barber HE. Plasma concentrations of edrophonium in man. *Clin Ther* 1976; **19:** 813–820

28. Kopman A. The pharmacokinetics of the anticholinesterase. *Anaesth Pharmacol Rev* 1993; **1:** 88–92

29. Hobbiger F. The mechanism of the anticholinesterase action of certain neostigmine analogues. *Br J Pharmacol* 1952; **7:** 223–236

30. Braga MFM, Rowan EG, Harvey AL & Bowman WC. Prejunctional action of neostigmine on mouse neuromuscular preparations. *Br J Anaesth* 1993; **70:** 405–410

31. Blaber LC. The mechanism of facilitatory action of edrophonium in cat skeletal muscle. *Br J Pharmacol* 1972; **46:** 498–503

32. Feldman SA. Discussion at 5th International Muscle Relaxant Meeting. Tokyo, Japan 1994

5

Neuromuscular block – non-depolarizing block

It is generally accepted that there are two types of neuromuscular block–non-depolarizing, competitive or antagonist block and depolarizing agonist block. Although it is appreciated that a reduction in neuromuscular transmission to the point of failure can be produced by other mechanisms such as depression of acetylcholine (ACh) synthesis (hemicholinium, etc.), storage (vesamicol, etc.) and release (magnesium, botulinus toxin, etc.), these mechanisms have not yet been widely exploited in clinical practice. Similarly, drugs that depress muscle activity such as dantrolene may be used for muscle relaxation but they are not neuromuscular blocking agents. When clinicians use the term neuromuscular block it therefore usually refers to either a depolarizing or a non-depolarizing block.

Non-depolarizing block results from competition between the antagonist drug and the neurotransmitter ACh for occupancy of the ACh recognition sites (AChR) on the α subunits of the receptor pentamer. This is a random competition between molecules of the agonist (ACh) and antagonist (in the form of a non-depolarizing blocking drug) and as such it obeys the law of mass action and the basic concept of competition.

This simplistic relationship indicates a general principle but in practice it is complicated by the finite number of receptors available and by the affinity constant of the drug with the receptor. The dissociation of the drug–receptor complex will free bound drug for more active competition, thus, although drugs with a low affinity can effectively increase their competitiveness by increased availability, drugs dissociating very slowly from a receptor will be more difficult to displace from a drug–receptor complex and will offer more effective and prolonged competition to ACh. As a result, the greater the affinity (the lower the K_D), the more effective is a drug as an antagonist and hence the more potent it will appear. The affinity of drugs is calculated from the Schild equation, usually presented as the Schild plot of the log dose–response to an agonist drug in the presence of different concentrations of antagonists (Fig. 5.1). In practice, this is usually determined by measuring the dose of agonist required to produce 50% twitch response in the presence of two concentrations of antagonist. It also follows that, in any equal mixture of antagonist drugs with a different K_D, the more potent drug (with the lower K_D) will appear to be most active and hence its effects will predominate.[1]

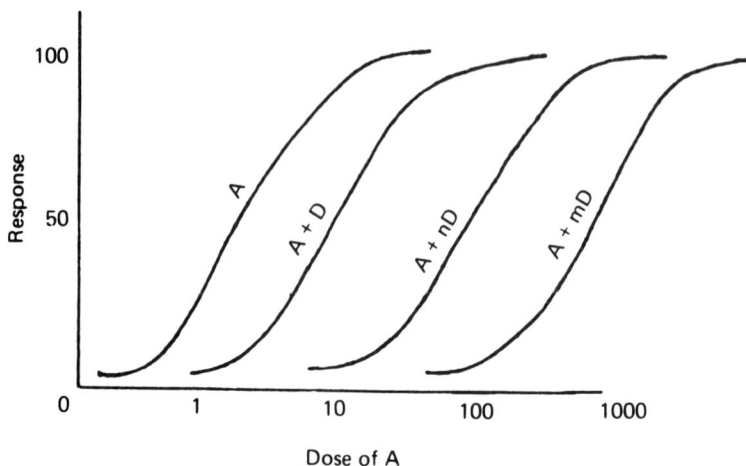

(a)

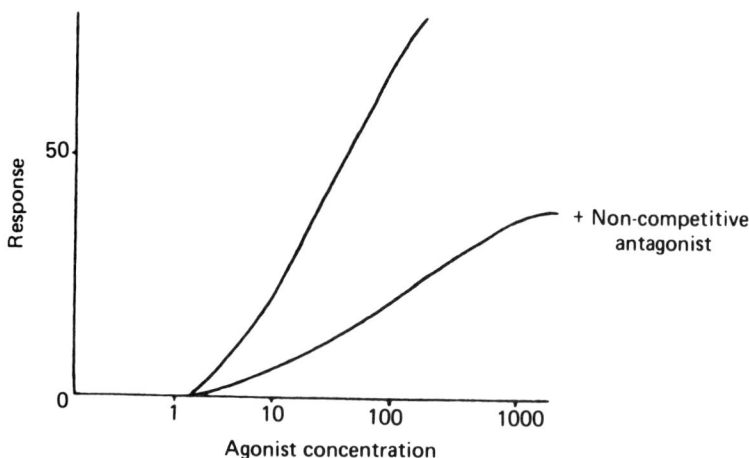

(b)

Fig. 5.1 (a) Schild plot showing parallel shift to the right to an agonist of log dose–response curves produced by increasing doses of antagonist. (b) Plot of a non-competitive agonist–antagonist relationship, demonstrating the flattening of response at high doses of antagonist.

The K_D of the presently used neuromuscular blocking drugs are all in the millisecond range and it follows that their effective action in the time scale of an operation or an experiment will be influenced by their concentration relative to that of ACh. Thus, washing out the drug from a reservoir *in vitro* without affecting the production of ACh reverses its action in a few minutes. Similarly, increasing the ACh concentration by means of an anticholinesterase should reduce the effect of the drug within a short period. This can be demonstrated in patch-clamp experiments where adding an agonist produces a microcurrent[2] within milliseconds – an effect which is abolished in milliseconds if an antagonist drug is introduced.[3,4] Once the drug is washed out, the agonist activity is rapidly re-established and the channel current can again be demonstrated.

Antagonist drugs such as tubocurare obey principles based on the law of mass action. If the concentration of drug relative to that of the agonist is kept constant (i.e. the effective blocking ratio of agonist to antagonist is kept constant), then the effect will be unchanged. In the presence of a higher dose of agonist it will be necessary to use an increased dose of antagonist to produce the same degree of block. Using increasing doses of antagonist and plotting the dose of agonist required to produce 25, 50 and 75% block in response to a given dose of agonist produces log dose–response curves. These should form a series of parallel lines (Fig. 5.1a). The slope of this line indicates the affinity constant of the drug and hence of its potency.

At higher concentrations of antagonist, however, the log dose–response curve loses its linearity and becomes flattened, resembling a non-competitive drug relationship (Fig. 5.1b). This has been attributed to a non-steady state or to a semi-equilibrium state[5] but, in spite of this oxymoronic term, it is difficult to explain this phenomenon when it occurs in an *in vitro* steady-state experiment where pharmacological equilibrium might be anticipated.

Since the receptor can be envisaged as either occupied by antagonist, by agonist or free of any drug, one can consider receptor occupancy in terms of drug concentration. The Hill plot of the receptor occupancy against log dose concentration of drug shows that the log of the ratio of receptors occupied by antagonist drug to free receptors is proportional to the log of the dose of drug administered if the concentration of agonist is unchanged. On a logit scale the receptor occupancy is linearly related to the log dose of drug.[6] As a result, it is possible to predict that doubling an ED_{50} dose of drug should produce 80% receptor occupancy and 10 times the ED_{50} dose will produce 91% receptor occupancy.[7]

The margin of safety

The concept of the margin of safety proposed by Paton and Waud in 1967[8] has greatly affected our understanding of events at the neuromuscular junction. Although the interpretation of their observations has recently been questioned (see Chapter 12), their results point to a requirement for non-depolarizing drugs to occupy a large number of drug receptor sites before the effect of competition with ACh produces depression of the twitch response. Paton and Waud estimated that a fractional occupancy of 78% of the available sites was required before antagonism of ACh produced depression of the twitch response and complete block occurred at 91% occupancy. These figures are similar to those calculated by Waser[9] from autoradiographic studies. Later studies by Waud and Waud[10] demonstrated that, at higher rates of stimulation, tetanic response was blocked at lower calculated levels of receptor occupancy (Fig. 5.2) and that at 100 Hz tetanic block occurred at about 50% receptor occlusion. The margin of safety concept allows us to consider different muscle sensitivity in terms of differing margins of safety.

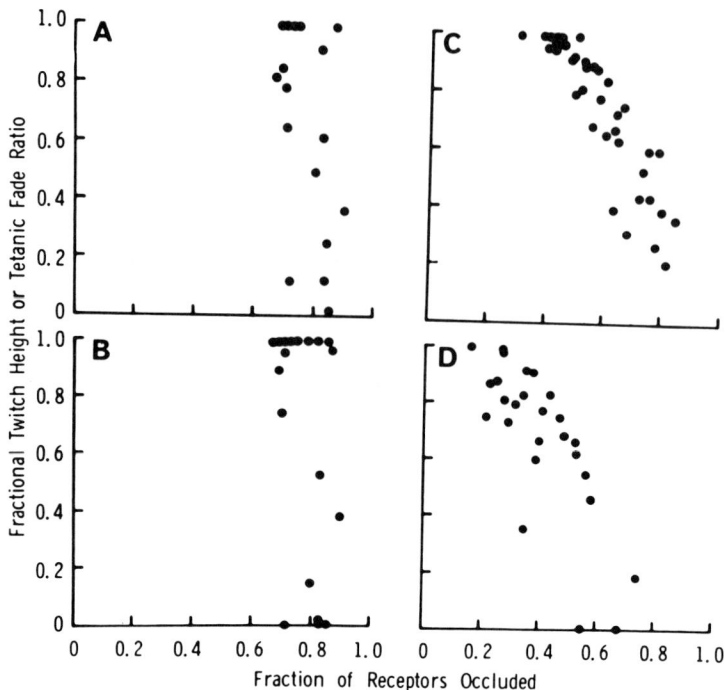

Fig 5.2 Effect of the rate of stimulation on the receptor occlusion fraction required to cause tetanic fade. A = 0.1 Hz; B = 30 Hz; C = 100 Hz; D = 200 Hz. From Waud and Waud.[10]

This is the basis of our understanding of the mechanism of non-depolarizing neuromuscular block. It is supported by studies in which drug or ACh is delivered into the neuromuscular junction using iontophoretic pulses through a micropipette. When an antagonist is administered, ACh is ineffective in producing an end-plate current. When it is washed out, the response to ACh is re-established. However, Armstrong and Lester reported that when tubocurare was used as the antagonist, the rate of onset of block was 10 times more rapid than recovery produced by the administration of ACh.[11] This suggests that the dissociation rate for tubo-curare was prolonged or some factor prevented its easy displacement from the receptor. Thus, in spite of a concentration gradient favourable to the removal of the antagonist from the synapse, its effect continued at a level that prevented the excess of ACh delivered by iontophoretic pulses from activating sufficient ACh receptors to produce a response (Fig. 5.3). They suggested that this effect might be due to the dense local concentration of receptors maintaining a high local level of drug in the synaptic cleft, pre-venting rapid reversal by ACh. They envisaged that tubocurare leaving one receptor would be restricted from diffusing away along its concentra-tion gradient and thus would be immediately available at a neighbouring receptor to increase the antagonist concentration at that site – an effect they termed buffered or restricted diffusion. This is rather like the local crowd effect that can be produced on a stage by the actors leaving on one

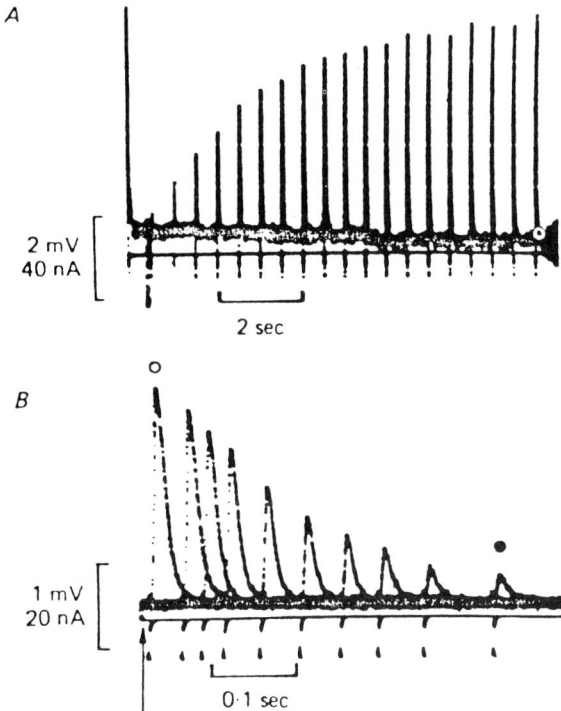

Fig. 5.3 The recovery from tubocurare block (trace A) has taken approximately 20 times as long as the onset of block (trace B) produced by iontophoretic pulses of antagonist. From Armstrong and Lester.[11]

side and reappearing on the other; by this means one actor (or drug molecule) can recirculate locally, producing a high local density, instead of dispersing into the wings of the theatre (or along the drug concentration gradient).

The basis of Armstrong and Lester's hypothesis was the observation that a small dose of α cobra venom reduced the recovery time by about 50%. They argued that this potent postsynaptic blocking drug reduced the density of ACh receptor population to a point where the effect was less marked and, as a result, the tubocurare molecules would be less restricted to the postsynaptic site. A small effect also occurred if the preparation was exposed to the action of a saponifying agent to destroy the Schwann cell membrane, suggesting that this membrane helped to restrict the phenomenon within the synaptic cleft. Various complex mathematical formulae based on unverifiable calculations of receptor sensitivity and speculative rate constants have been devised to support this hypothesis; however, none explains why this effect is not seen with depolarizing drugs whose charge density is in the same order as that of tubocurare. Observations in humans with decamethonium suggest that the rate of spontaneous recovery is almost as rapid as onset if the drug concentration gradient is similar. Although buffered diffusion has not been demonstrated with any agent other than tubocurare, the observations of Armstrong and Lester[11] drew attention to the fact that at the microlevel of synaptic cleft, something occurs that modifies the relationship between the extrasynaptic concentration of drug and the amount of block. Their finding that, in spite of an excess of ACh, it takes 10 times longer to reverse the tubocurare block than would have been expected had the free ingress of drug molecules underlying onset been matched by the egress of the tubocurare during recovery, necessitates modifying the concept of simple competion kinetics in order to understand events occurring at the receptor. Since there is no evidence to suggest that tubocurare enters muscle or is partitioned in any tissue, it points to a binding mechanism for the drug molecules within the synapse. Since the affinity of tubocurare for the ACh receptor itself is calculated to be in the millisecond range, it is necessary to invoke some additional mechanism to explain the slow reversal. Buffered diffusion is one of the suggestions as to how this may occur.

In 1970 Feldman and Tyrrell[12] presented a paper describing a phenomenon in patients similar to that later described in single muscle fibres by Armstrong and Lester. Following the use of a small dose of tubocurare (3 mg) with local anaesthetic in a series of Bier's blocks in order to relieve muscle spasm, Feldman and Tyrrell noticed that upon release of the tourniquet there was rapid return of sensation as the local anaesthetic effect wore off, but that the return of motor power often took up to an hour. As a result, experiments were performed using various neuromuscular blocking drugs in the isolated arm; these confirmed that, following release of the tourniquet, 3 min after administering 40 ml of saline containing a small dose of the drug (20% of an ED_{90}), recovery of twitch response took up to 60 min depending upon the drug studied. Feldman and Tyrrell postulated that a mechanism must exist for binding non-depolarizing drugs at the receptor site and that this was not shared by the depolarizing drug decamethonium (C_{10}).[12,13]

This suggestion was supported by a series of experiments which confirmed that the primary rate-limiting condition for the recovery of non-depolarizing neuromuscular block was the dissociation of drug from these binding sites and this rate varied according to the drug used.[11,12] It was demonstrated that the effect of the drug in the plasma is secondary to this effect; a higher plasma level of drug further delayed recovery from the block[15] (Figs 5.4 and 5.5).

In 1974, Matteo et al.[16] described a radioimmunoassay technique that allowed the plasma concentration of tubocurare to be accurately assayed. Using this methodology they demonstrated that, following administration of tubocurare, the plasma concentration of drug diminished as the neuromuscular block recovered. They suggested that the relationship between plasma concentration of drug and degree of neuromuscular block proved this cause and effect and that recovery of neuromuscular function was the direct result of the plasma clearance of drug. This interpretation was questioned, and it was pointed out that it was unlikely that the block would not decrease with time and that the plasma level of drug would invariably fall, but this casual association of these events did not prove a cause and effect relationship.[17] This was the beginning of pharmacokinetic modelling based upon the concept that it is the plasma level of drug that determines

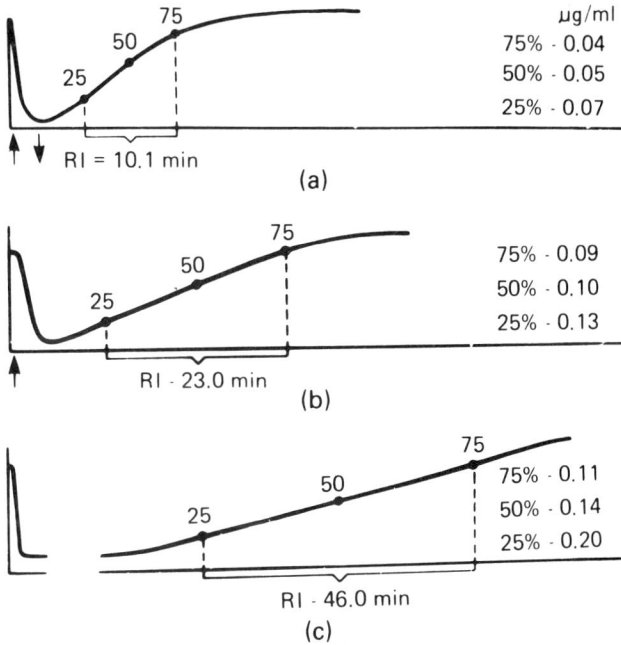

	µg/ml
75%	0.04
50%	0.05
25%	0.07

RI = 10.1 min

(a)

75%	0.09
50%	0.10
25%	0.13

RI - 23.0 min

(b)

75%	0.11
50%	0.14
25%	0.20

RI - 46.0 min

(c)

Fig. 5.4 Recovery rate and plasma concentration of pancuronium (a) in the isolated arm; (b) bolus injection; (c) after continuous infusion. The higher the plasma concentration of the drug the slower the recovery.

the degree of block. This interpretation fails to take into account the importance of biophase events that Feldman and Tyrrell[12] and Armstrong and Lester[11] demonstrated may modify the rate of onset and offset of neuromuscular block. Only in a state of equilibrium will the events in the biophase and in the plasma correspond and the events modelled from plasma concentrations of drug reflect the amount of block. In the conditions occurring in clinical practice, with rapidly declining plasma levels of drug, it is the biophase component, revealed in the isolated arm studies

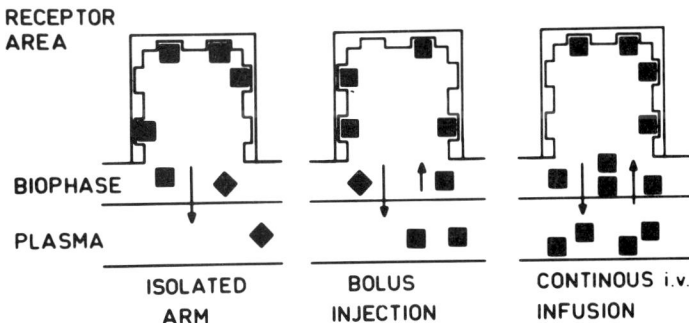

RECEPTOR AREA

BIOPHASE

PLASMA

ISOLATED ARM   BOLUS INJECTION   CONTINOUS i.v. INFUSION

Fig. 5.5 How it is envisaged that the plasma concentration of drug inhibits recovery from neuromuscular block by reducing the synaptic cleft–plasma concentration gradient. From Agoston et al.,[14] with permission.

and in the studies of Armstrong and Lester, that determines the degree of neuromuscular block.[18]

Since the events occurring in the biophase are the primary determinants of the recovery rate of neuromuscular blocking drugs, it is sensible to understand this process. The principal method of study of this phenomenon has been the isolated arm and isolated forearm experiments. Many of the results of these studies correspond to the effect seen following close intra-arterial injection of a small dose of drug with temporary venous occlusion. As most human investigations have been performed by the Westminster group using the isolated arm and forearm, it is useful to review these studies (see Chapter 6).

References

1. Ginsberg BL & Stephenson RP. On the simultaneous action of two competitive antagonists. *Br J Pharmol* 1974; **51**: 287–300
2. Colquhoun D & Sackman B. Fluctuations in the microsecond time range of the current through single acetylcholine receptor ion channels. *Nature* 1981; **294**: 464–466
3. Colquhoun D & Sheridan RE. The effect of tubocurarine competition on the kinetics of agonist action on the nicotinic receptor. *Br J Pharmacol* 1982; **75**: 77–86
4. Colquhoun D. (1986) On the principles of postsynaptic action of neuromuscular blocking agents. In: *New Neuromuscular Blocking Agents. Handbook of Experimental Pharmacology*. Kharkevicy DS (ed.). Berlin: Springer Verlag, pp. 59–113
5. Waud BE & Waud D. (1990) Muscle relaxant interactions. In: *Muscle Relaxants*. Agoston S & Bowman WC (eds). Holland: Elsevier Science, pp. 231–243
6. Norman J. (1984) Drug receptor reactions. In: *Pharmacokinetics of Anaesthesia*. Prys-Roberts C & Hug CC (eds). Oxford: Oxford Scientific Publishers, pp. 25–37
7. Bevan DR, Bevan C & Donati R. (1988) Pharmacokinetic principles. In: *Muscle Relaxants in Clinical Anaesthesia*. London: Year Book, pp. 100–128
8. Paton WDM & Waud DR. The margin of safety of neuromuscular transmission. *J Physiol* 1967; **191**: 50–90
9. Waser PG. (1990) On receptors in the post-synaptic membrane at the motor end plate. In: *CIBA Foundation Symposium on Molecular Properties of Drug Receptors*. Porter R & O'Connor M (eds). London: Churchill, p. 59
10. Waud DR & Waud BE. The relation between tetanic fade and receptor occlusion in the presence of competitive neuromuscular block. *Anesthesiology* 1971; **35**: 456–461
11. Armstrong DL & Lester HA. The kinetics of tubocurarine action and restricted diffusion. *J Physiol* 1979; **294**: 365–376
12. Feldman SA & Tyrrell MF. A new theory of the termination of action of the muscle relaxants. *Proc R Soc Med* 1970; **63**: 692–694
13. Feldman SA. Affinity concept and the action of the muscle relaxants. *Acta Anesthesiol Belg* 1976; **27**: 86–96
14. Feldman S. Biophase binding: its effect on recovery from non depolarizing neuromuscular block. *Anaesthesiol Pharmacol Rev* 1993; **1**: 81–87
15. Agoston S, Feldman S & Miller RD. Plasma pancuronium and twitch response using the isolated arm, following bolus injection and continuous infusion. *Anesthesiology* 1979, **51**: 119–123
16. Matteo RS, Spector S & Horrowitz PE. Relation of serum *d*-tubocurarine to neuromuscular blockade in man. *Anesthesiology* 1974; **41**: 440–443
17. Feldman SA. Serum dTc and neuromuscular blockade in man. *Anesthesiology* 1975; **42**: 644–645
18. Campkin NTA & Hood JR. The isolated arm. *Anaesthesiol Pharmacol Rev* 1993; **1**: 77–80

6

Isolated arm experiments

Much of the evidence presented to support the views in this book is predicated on experiments carried out in the isolated arm or isolated forearm. It is sensible, therefore, to consider the nature of these experiments in some detail so that one can better appreciate the meaningfulness of the results.

The concept was provoked by the necessity to provide more suitable surgical conditions for the reduction of Colles fractures carried out under Bier's block. The block produces adequate conditions in the elderly but in younger, more muscular patients, it is often difficult to obtain sufficient muscle relaxation with local anaesthetic alone. During the winter of 1961–62 the author began adding 2–3 mg of tubocurare to the 0.5% lignocaine then in widespread use. It was noticeable that upon release of tourniquet, at the end of the procedure, motor power remained poor in the arm long after the sensation of pain had returned.

Initial experiments using a sphygmomanometer bulb in the hand attached to a mercury manometer to test for muscle weakness demonstrated that it took up to 45 min for motor power to return and that, even then, fine muscle movement was difficult for up to 30 min more. These experiments were carried out with Dr John Hoyle but the results were difficult to quantify and were not published. Tyrrell,[1] using a Statham UC3 Gold Cell, designed a more suitable apparatus to transduce the force of contraction of the adductor pollicis muscles. Adequately controlled experiments were carried out. The first series of results on which the present theory is partially based were published in 1970.[2]

Other workers have also used similar techniques for other purposes, notably Torda and Klonymus, who also advocated the addition of a small dose of relaxant into the Bier's block to reduce muscle tone,[3] as well as Foldes.[4] Foldes recommended its use as a potential test for myasthenics and we have confirmed its usefulness for this purpose when in the absence of receptor antibodies a myasthenic state is present, usually due to glandular dysfunction.

The isolated arm technique

A sphygmomanometer cuff is placed on the arm selected for the experiment (Fig. 6.1). An indwelling needle is placed in a vein on the dorsum of

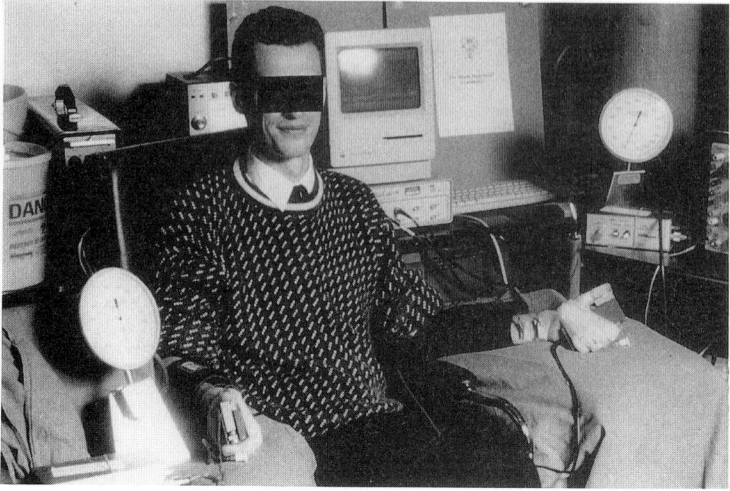

Fig. 6.1 The isolated arm (forearm) experiment.

the hand and a suitable strain gauge is fixed in the hand to measure the force of contraction of the adductor pollicis muscles. We presently use an RS 2G strain gauge modified with an adjustable cradle to allow fixation of the thumb. This gives a linear response suitable for twitch measurements. A similar arrangement using a 20G strain gauge is used to transduce the force of tetanic contraction. The thumb should be extended as close to 90° to the hand as is convenient and the cradle adjusted to give a preloading tension of between 200 and 300G. The preload ensures a similar degree of isotonicity in similar experiments. The ulnar nerve was stimulated in the initial experiments through subcutaneous fine-needle electrodes placed longitudinally over the ulnar nerve at the wrist. In the present series of experiments we have used silver–silver chloride surface electrodes. The stimulation voltage must be supramaximal to ensure that all muscle fibres that can respond are stimulated at all times. It is usual to find that a voltage of 90–110 V with a pulse width no greater than 0.2 ms is required. Recommended stimulation rates vary but we have found a twitch stimulation of 0.2 Hz satisfactory to allow us to follow rapidly changing events, in the onset of block, as well as the slower recovery. Other authors have recommended slower rates, but these are too slow to allow cumulative log dose–response effects to be monitored during onset.

Once the apparatus is in position, a period of 5–10 min is allowed for stabilization, the tourniquet is then inflated to 280–300 mmHg and the drug under test, diluted in 40 ml of saline, is immediately injected into the indwelling needle over 60 s. It is noticeable that venous distension occurs and occasionally this provokes some discomfort. As the drug passes from the distended veins retrograde into the capillaries it is not uncommon to feel 'pins and needles' and itching, especially if a benzyl-isoquinolinium drug is used. Neuromuscular block starts to occur within 30 s and is usually complete in 3–5 min. In the initial series of experiments approximately 10% (i.e. 20% of the ED_{90}) of the clinical bolus dose of drug was used and the tourniquet was deflated in 3 min. With this dose it is not uncommon for some diplopia to be noticed, when the tourniquet is released, this lasts for about 5 min.

With all the non-depolarizing drugs studied there is a slow recovery from neuromuscular block in spite of the rapid decline in plasma concentration of drug that must occur once the tourniquet is released and arterial blood, free of drug, once again perfuses the arm. The recovery index (RI) is taken as a measure of the rate of recovery. This is the time taken for the twitch response to recover from 25 to 75% of initial control. This slow recovery, in the presence of a rapid decline in plasma concentration of drug, led Feldman and Tyrrell[2] in 1970 to postulate binding of the drug to the receptor. A typical trace is shown in Figure 6.2.

Using the middle half of the recovery slope to make measurements of recovery rates avoids distortions that could be caused by a non-linear start to recovery and a slowing-down once greater than 75% recovery had been obtained. It is invariably less than 50% of the time from 5 to 95% recovery. The RI for the non-depolarizing drugs varies between 7 and 20 min; it is different for each drug and generally bears a direct relationship to the RI following bolus injection of an ED_{95} dose. Thus, the short-acting drugs such as mivacurium and vecuronium have a shorter RI than pancuronium, tubocurare and doxacurium (Table 6.1).

Feldman and Tyrrell also demonstrated that depolarizing drugs such as decamethonium (C_{10}) duration of action 15–20 min following bolus systemic ED_{95} dose) have a rapid RI in the isolated arm which more closely resembles a washout of drug (Fig. 6.3). They postulated that, unlike non-depolarizing drugs, C_{10} was not bound to the receptor or in the biophase.

It is an interesting observation that, whilst the arm is paralysed, the pain of the stimulation is greatly diminished and the fingers lose acuity of sensation. It has been suggested that this is the result of paralysis of muscle spindle input to the brain from the arm and hand.

Control experiments have demonstrated that occlusion of the circulation to the arm for up to 6 min does not affect subsequent neuromuscular block and that following release of the tourniquet, even after 3 min, causes blood

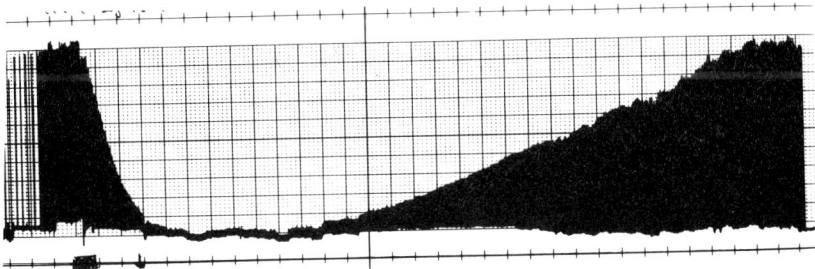

Fig. 6.2 The isolated arm experiment. Vecuronium 0.6 mg in 40 ml saline was injected at ■ and the tourniquet released 2 min later. The duration of recovery from 25 to 75% twitch height was 8.4 min.

Table 6.1 Time taken from 25 to 75% recovery of twitch response using various drugs

Drug	Recovery index (min)
Gallamine	9.8
Tubocurare	12.8
Vecuronium	9.3
Pancuronium	14.2
Pipecuronium	10.8
Atracurium	9.5
Mivacurium	8.4
Doxacurium	18.3

Results were obtained from published data in different experiments carried out at different times.

flow to be considerably increased and the onset time of a subsequent block to be somewhat decreased.

There can be little doubt that the events observed represent the effect of the spread of fluid-containing drug from the distended veins into the capillary bed and hence into the ECF and synaptic cleft (Fig. 6.4). In this way its effects are the same as giving a small dose of drug by close intra-arterial injection during a short period of venous occlusion. The results of intra-arterial and isolated arm injections are similar.

Whilst venous back-pressure remains there will be a driving force encouraging drug to pass into the extracellular fluid and into the synaptic cleft. Once the tourniquet is released the pressure gradient will be reversed as fresh arterial blood floods into the system driving out any residue of drug into the systemic circulation. It is this recirculating drug that produces the transient diplopia. If a larger volume is used or if it is too forcibly injected, petechial haemorrhage may occur, indicating the effect of excessive back-pressure on the capillary system.

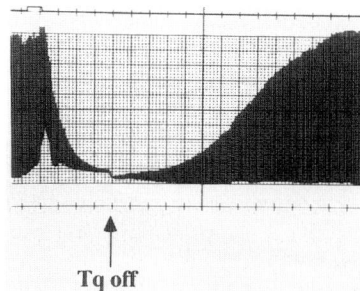

Tq off

Fig. 6.3 Decamethonium in the isolated arm. The recovery of the twitch response is rapid, suggesting that the drug is not bound but is easily washed out of the synaptic cleft. TQ = Tourniquet.

Vein

Artery   ECF

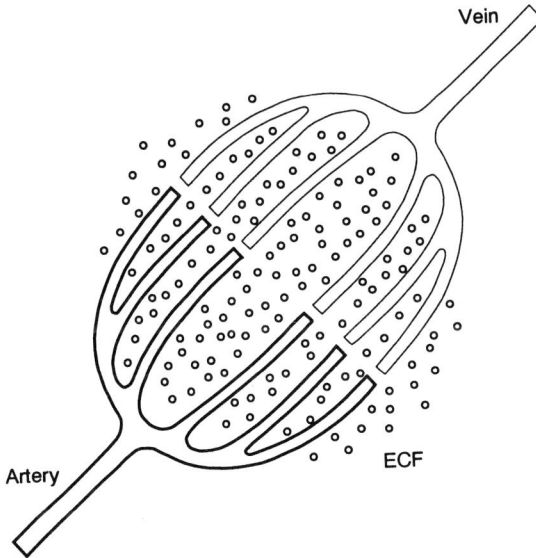

Fig. 6.4 The isolated arm or forearm experiment distends the venous capillary bed, forcing drug into the extracellular fluid (ECF). It is analogous to administering a similar dose of drug by close intra-arterial injection and temporarily occluding the venous outflow.

The isolated forearm

In the more recent series of experiments we have modified the technique by placing the isolating tourniquet on the forearm. We have selected doses of drugs that produce about 95% block in 3 min tourniquet time (usually about 10% of the ED_{90} dose). As only the forearm veins are involved, a smaller quantity of diluent saline is used (20 ml saline as opposed to 40 ml). One of the advantages of this isolated arm technique is that it is possible to study two different drugs in the two arms of volunteers simultaneously as the dose of drug used in each arm is reduced by about 50% compared to that used in the isolated arm (Figs 6.5 and 6.6).

Although a great effort is made to control all possible variables, such as the temperature of the arm and injection fluid, it is nevertheless puzzling that the same volunteer may demonstrate up to a 25% variability in recovery using the same drug and from the same degree of block in different studies. However, when two different drugs are used in the two arms a more rapid recovery from one drug is usually accompanied by a more rapid recovery from the other drug in the opposite forearm, so that the relationship between recovery times is fairly constant. On only two occasions in more than 100 experiments has this relationship not been maintained. The reason for the variability of the results is not readily apparent and it may represent a biological fluctuation in receptor sensitivity from day to day. It may be the cause of the variations in the RI (time from recovery from 25 to 75% of the twitch response) reported in the various series of experiments. An additional possible contributing

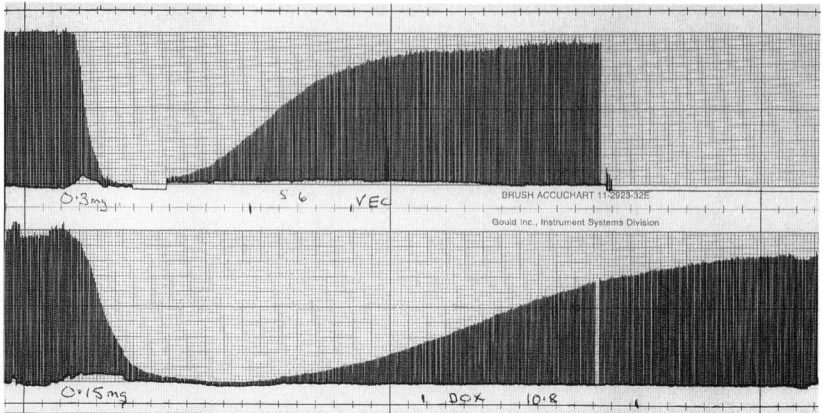

Fig. 6.5 Simultaneous administration of vecuronium 0.3 mg (upper trace) in one isolated forearm and doxacurium 0.15 mg (lower trace) in the other.

factor may be the use of different drugs in the contralateral arm. It is theoretically possible that the small amount of circulating drugs released when the tourniquet is deflated may influence the recovery in the forearms by displacing less avidly bound drug. However, the cause of this biological variation is most probably associated with the position of the venous access site and the distending pressure established when the drug is injected, as this may well influence the proportion of injectate that reaches the adductor pollicis muscle.

One of the interesting observations made using the bilateral isolated arm experiment which emphasizes the difficulty of explaining the findings without postulating a binding of drug came from the cross-over experiments.[5] In these experiments pancuronium was administered to one

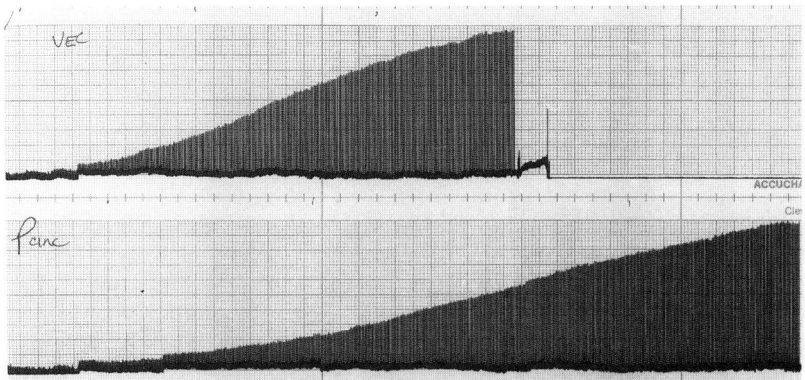

Fig. 6.6 Results from simultaneously administering vecuronium 0.3 mg (top) into one forearm of a volunteer, whilst pancuronium 0.3 mg (bottom) was given in the other. Different recovery indices are found, in spite of both arms being perfused by blood containing the same small content of both drugs once the tourniquet was released.

isolated forearm in volunteers whilst vecuronium was given in the other. At 50% recovery of the twitch response the tourniquet was reinflated and pancuronium administered to the arm that had received vecuronium and vecuronium to the arm recovering from pancuronium. It was found that the second drug now recovered at a rate more like the first drug, i.e. vecuronium recovery was prolonged while that of pancuronium was reduced (Fig. 6.7). The ability of the original drug to affect recovery of the second drug is most readily interpreted as being the result of the reservoir of the first drug still being present bound in the biophase when the second administration was made.

The effect in the isolated arm is reflected in the findings following systemic bolus doses of drugs in patients during anaesthesia. Thus, mivacurium given immediately after pancuronium has a longer than expected duration of action.

Pharmacokinetics of the isolated arm and forearm

It has proved difficult to obtain information about the pharmacokinetics of the isolated arm experiments due to the very low concentrations of drug in the plasma following release of the tourniquet and the impossibility of measuring directly how much drug remains in the arm and in what compartment it resides. As a result, much of the information has been conjectural and as such open to alternative explanations.

It appears likely that water-soluble drugs such as the neuromuscular blocking agents will rapidly be distributed in the extracellular fluid and the synaptic cleft as the Schwann cell membrane does not appear to offer a significant barrier to these drugs (see Chapter 9). Similarly, it is difficult to envisage a barrier to the washout of these drugs along their concentration gradient once the tourniquet is released. To speculate where drug may be sequestrated in the short period of exposure (it can be as brief as 10 s) necessitates postulating either a barrier to egress of the drug but not to ingress (such as is postulated in the theory of buffered diffusion), the penetration of drug into cells such as muscle where it remains as a reservoir or binding to non-specific acceptor sites. There is no evidence that

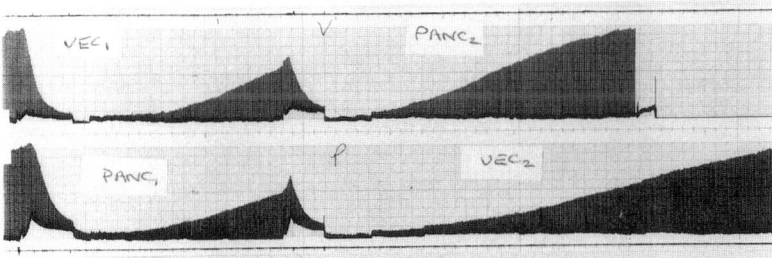

Fig. 6.7 The cross-over experiment. Vecuronium was administered in one isolated forearm whilst pancuronium was given in the other. At 50% recovery the drugs were crossed over and the experiment repeated. The block from the second drug now recovers at a rate influenced by the first.

non-depolarizing drugs enter muscle, although depolarizing drugs such as C_{10} may do so. There is autoradiographic evidence of drug being trapped in the synaptic cleft and that this drug is associated with the receptor substance itself or with cholinesterase (Fig. 6.8). If non-specific partitioning, as suggested by Sheiner et al.[6] and Stanski and Sheiner,[8] did occur it should be greatest with drugs such as C_{10} which can be demonstrated to enter muscle, albeit slowly, and for more fat-soluble drugs such as vecuronium in comparison   to the less fat-soluble pancuronium. In fact, evidence from the isolated arm suggests that the reverse occurs. There is rapid recovery from C_{10} block and the recovery from pancuronium in the isolated arm is slower than vecuronium.

In an effort to settle the controversy we have studied the pharmacokinetics of atracurium in the isolated forearm and compared it to labelled ethylenediaminetetraacetic acid (EDTA). Before the release of the tourniquet the concentration of atracurium in a large vein in the isolated forearm (some distance from the site of injection on the back of the hand) was in the region of 800 ng/ml. There was evidence of a slow decline in this concentration, possibly due to a small leak from under the tourniquet in the isolated forearm. Following release of the tourniquet the plasma concentration fell rapidly, producing a washout curve, and the plasma concentrates reached 10–40 ng/ml in the venous blood of both the blocked arm and the contralateral arm in 5 min (Fig. 6.9). The washout curve for atracurium was the same as that found with EDTA. It is evident that, following release of the tourniquet, atracurium behaves as predicted for a water-soluble drug and that there is no significant non-specific partitioning in the tissues, as proposed by pharmacokinetic models. It is clear that the reservoir of drug necessary to cause the slow reversal of drug action must be small, finite and related to local acceptor binding sites. It is also unlikely that the very low level of plasma atracurium found after release of the tourniquet plays a role in prolonging the action of the drug, causing the slow recovery we have observed.

(a)   (b)

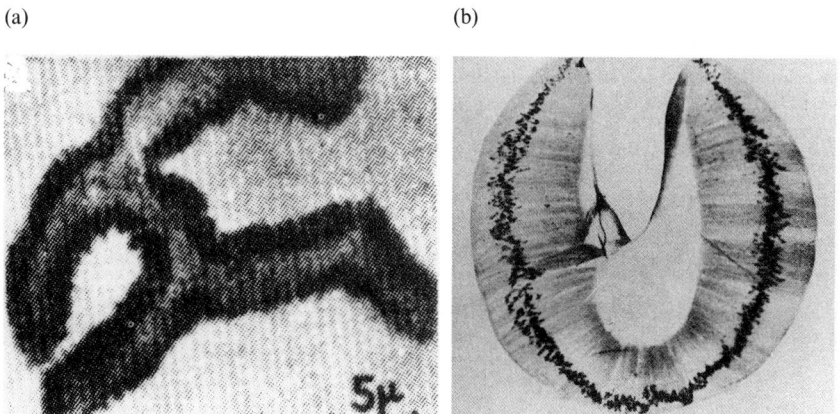

Fig. 6.8 (a) Autoradiographic evidence of C_{14}-labelled toxiferine still present in the synaptic cleft after repeated washings. From Conteaux and Taxi 1968. (b) Autoradiographic evidence of curare retained at the neuromuscular junction in rat diaphragms in spite of repeated washings. From Waser 1969.

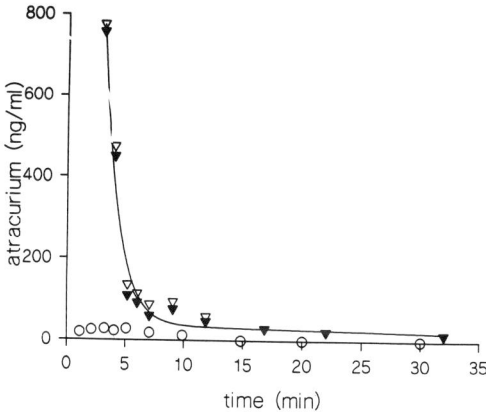

Fig. 6.9 The washout of drug (▽) or ethylenediaminetetraacetic acid (EDTA) (▼) in the isolated forearm on release of the tourniquet at 5 min, compared to background drug concentration in plasma (○).

Interpretation of results

The isolated arm and forearm is used principally to study recovery from neuromuscular block although it can also be used to compare onset times if special precautions are taken. Because the dose of drug used is small, especially in the isolated forearm experiments, the recovery observed occurs whilst the plasma concentration of drug is declining from an already very low (often unmeasurable) level following release of the tourniquet. It is therefore reasonable to interpret the time from 25 to 75% recovery of the twitch height as indicating the spontaneous recovery rate of neuromuscular transmission uninfluenced by pharmacokinetic effects. These conditions are analogous to those in a water bath after removing the drug and washing the preparation or after a small local intra-arterial injection of drug. The finding that the spontaneous recovery rates of different drugs vary in the absence of significant drug in the plasma led to the assertion in 1970 that they are subject to physicochemical forces that bind them to the receptor.[2] At that time the anatomy of the receptor pentamer was unknown. It is unlikely that molecules of a drug are bound to the acetylcholine (ACh) receptor itself although it has been demonstrated that the affinity of the two ACh receptors for tubocurare differs 100-fold, it is still too low to account for the prolonged effect observed in these experiments. In the present state of our knowledge it is therefore difficult to come to any conclusion, other than that some physicochemical force binds these drugs in the effect compartment or biophase.

A less valuable measurement that can be made in the isolated arm experiment is the time from release of the tourniquet to 25% recovery of the twitch response. This measurement more closely indicates the quantity of the block than the rate of recovery. Generally the 0–25% recovery time will increase with increasing dose of drug administered in the 20 ml of saline in the isolated forearm. However, we have found that increasing the dose from 0.3 to 0.5 mg in the isolated forearm increased the mean 0–25% recovery time (in volunteers) more than increasing it from 0.5 to 2.0 mg (in anaesthetized patients). Even after 1.5 mg in the isolated forearm, the 0–25% recovery time seldom exceeds 10 min in anaesthetized patients. This suggests that the binding potential of the biophase is finite and saturable. Even at high doses where the plasma level after release of the tourniquet would be expected to play a significant role there is little evidence of a large extension of this binding capacity, indicated by the 0–25% recovery time, beyond that produced by more modest doses of drugs.

It is proposed therefore that the isolated arm, and more particularly the bilateral isolated forearm experiments, where a control drug can be tested against another drug in the opposite arm, provides evidence of the relative affinity of the relaxants with biophase binding sites. These binding sites are readily saturable. It provides an opportunity to study the spontaneous rate of recovery of a drug uninfluenced or affected only to an insignificant degree by the changing concentration of drug in the plasma and by pharmacokinetic events. As such it is a valuable experimental tool and an excellent test bed for new drugs.

The isolated arm experiments gave rise to the concept, expressed in their paper by Feldman and Tyrrell in 1970,[2] that the pharmacodynamics and behaviour of a drug in the biophase primarily determined the rate of recovery from neuromuscular block following a bolus injection of drug.[9,10] A further study suggested that the influence of the plasma concentration of drug was secondary and acted to reduce the concentration gradient between biophase and plasma which is maximized in the isolated arm experiment. In this study by Agoston and colleagues,[11] it was found that the recovery was slowest when the plasma concentration of drug was highest. It was quickest in the isolated arm experiments where the gradient between the synaptic cleft and plasma was highest as the concentration of drug in the blood was very low.[11] Only in steady-state conditions, where the drug concentration gradient between the plasma and biophase is minimal, do pharmacokinetic influences control the rate of recovery of the block (see Chapter 5).

At about the same time as this theory was being developed, more reliable methods of estimating the concentration of the relaxants were being developed to supplement the old difficult spectrofluorometric methodology of Pittanger et al.[12] Cohen et al.[13] developed an H^3-labelled method of analysing plasma concentrations of tubocurare and gallamine, and Matteo and associates[14] developed a radioimmune analysis of tubocurare. They used this method to demonstrate that, following bolus injection of tubocurare, the plasma level fell and the twitch height recovered. Although this result was to be expected – indeed, a contrary finding would have been impossible to explain – it was taken to indicate a causal relationship between the reduction in plasma concentration of drug and recovery of neuromuscular conduction. This was the beginning of pharmacokinetics and computer modelling. Within 5 years, incomprehensibly complex models had been developed to explain the relationship between plasma concentration and effect. However, as all the models started with data obtained from clinical measurements, they were at best a derived form of presenting information and to suggest that they in any way conferred validity upon the original assumption that the plasma level alone determined recovery from neuromuscular block in a non-steady state was making an unwarranted assumption.

However, as the biophase binding concept conflicted with the assumptions of the pharmacokineticists, it remained for the advocates of the kinetic theory to explain the findings of the isolated arm experiments. The suggestions made include the following:

1 The neuromuscular block in the isolated arm experiments in some way differed from 'normal neuromuscular block'.
2 The results in the isolated arm can be explained in terms of muscle perfusion.[18]
3 The results represent partitioning of the drug.[8]
4 The results are due to recirculation of drug in the plasma.[9]

1. Type of block

As far as is known, once a neuromuscular blocking drug is introduced into the synaptic cleft in sufficient concentration to reduce the effectiveness of ACh, it will produce block of the nicotinic receptors irrespective of the manner by which it was administered. This may be by diffusion through the tissues of the diaphragm in a water bath, following close intra-arterial injection, intravenous injection or following retrograde venous spread in the isolated arm. There is no evidence that the block produced in the isolated arm causing 95% depression of the twitch is 'overwhelmingly massively overdosed' or in any way different from that seen in clinical practice.

2. Blood flow

Waud[15] and Stanski and Sheiner,[8] in an effort to explain the slow offset of block found in the isolated arm following tubocurare block, suggested that it was to be expected on the basis of the low blood flow to resting muscle and hence the time required to achieve clearance of drug from the muscle. The blood flow to muscle varies by 300–400% depending upon type of muscle and state of activity.[17] The blood flow to the neuromuscular junction has not been well-studied but is derived from the arterial supply to the motor nerve. The clearance of drug from the neuromuscular junction is unknown but recovery from neuromuscular block does not appear to be seriously prolonged in conditions of reduced flow[18] and low muscle blood flow, although there is evidence that at very low perfusion rates, tissue hypoxia may prolong recovery. Certainly it has been clearly demonstrated that increasing blood flow to muscle by up to eight times the control flow does not alter the rate of recovery of non-depolarizing neuromuscular block,[19,20] even if the perfusing blood contains no drug.[21] It therefore appears unlikely that muscle blood flow is the limiting factor in the recovery from neuromuscular block in the isolated arm after tubocurare.

Conclusive evidence that muscle blood flow does not prevent a faster recovery of block than is seen with tubocurare is provided by the finding that C_{10} block recovers five times faster than that following tubocurare in the isolated arm and that the RI of vecuronium is much quicker than pancuronium when one drug is administered to one forearm and the other to the contralateral arm. It is inconceivable that the arm receiving the vecuronium would have a more rapid muscle blood flow than the opposite forearm that had been blocked by pancuronium.

3. Partitioning of drug

The term partitioning usually refers to the differences in the concentration of drug in different tissues, resulting from the physical properties of that drug such as solubility, electrostatic charge, etc. However, all the relaxant drugs have similar physical properties and would be expected to have similar partitioning characteristics. Stanski, in a well-reasoned editorial, suggested that partitioning of drug in the tissue of the neuromuscular junction might account for the slow recovery from neuromuscular block in the isolated arm.[7] Apart from the difficulty of explaining why C_{10}, the one drug which has been demonstrated to partition easily into muscle, recovers more rapidly than all non-depolarizing drugs, partitioning fails to explain where the drug goes. All the neuromuscular blocking drugs are water-soluble and readily pass into the extracellular water but none can be readily demonstrated in tissues around the neuromuscular junction.

The only evidence that these drugs appear to be partitioned comes from autoradiography which clearly shows radioactive drug associated with the postsynaptic secondary clefts, where the receptors are known to be congregated (Fig. 6.8a). With the exception of C_{10} and possibly gallamine, none of the neuromuscular blocking drugs appears to pass into the muscle in a manner that could be accepted as partitioning. Waser and his coworkers[27] measured the redistribution of C_{14}-labelled vecuronium in rats and mice and measured the radioactivity appearing in muscle, including the neuromuscular junction. They found that the highest concentration reached in muscle was a fraction of that in the liver, kidney and blood (Fig. 6.10). Partitioning also fails to explain the very different rates of recovery in the isolated forearms of two closely related drugs such as vecuronium and pancuronium (Fig. 6.6). Both drugs have a similar molecular size charge and, of the two drugs, it is vecuronium that is slightly more fat-soluble and therefore a more likely candidate for partitioning in muscle, yet vecuronium has a more rapid RI.

Recirculation of drugs in plasma

Hull[16] offered an alternative explanation of the unexpectedly slow recovery from tubocurare neuromuscular block in the isolated arm. He noted the short sensation of diplopia following release of the tourniquet and reasoned that it signified a sufficient residual plasma concentration of drug to slow the rate of washout of drug from the biophase. He pointed out the frequent small increases in neuromuscular block that occurred as soon as the tourniquet was released and suggested that this might be due

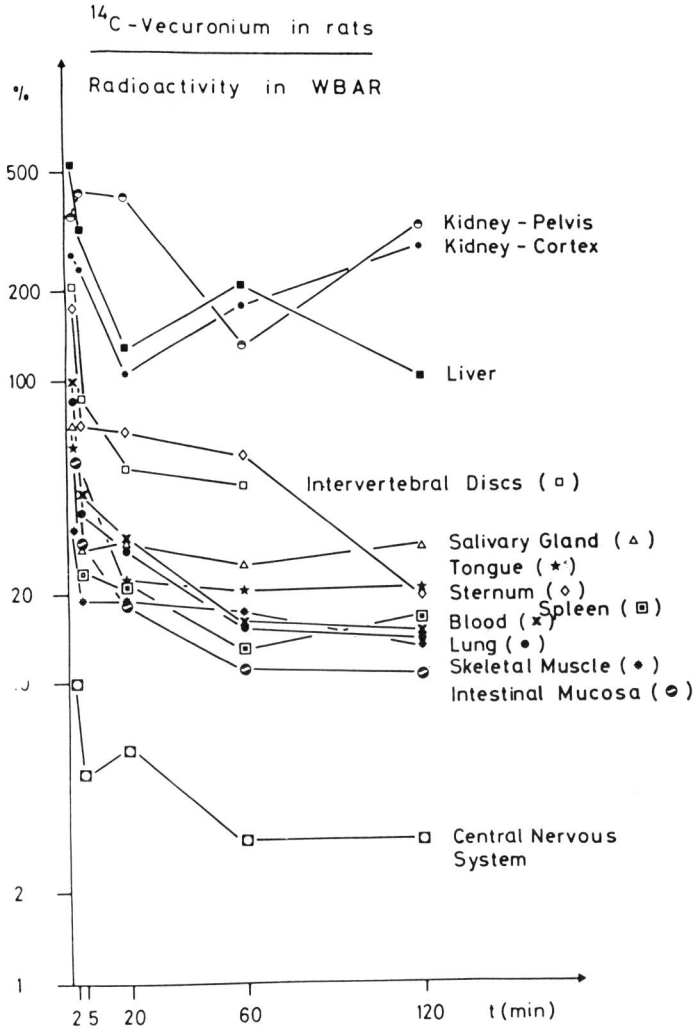

Fig. 6.10 Concentrations of C_{14} vecuronium in various rat tissues. Note the low concentration in muscle. From Waser et al.[27]

to a short-lived surge in plasma drug concentration. By applying the dose of drug administered in the isolated arm to a complex model proposed for the pharmacodynamics of fazadinium and pancuronium, he purported to prove that this explanation was tenable.

Little effort has been made to measure the plasma drug concentrations following release of the tourniquet in the isolated arm, as the concentrations are so low that they are extremely difficult to measure with any degree of certainty. However, the research unit at Groningen University did measure the plasma concentration after 0.6 mg of pancuronium was administered into the isolated arm and found it to be in the subclinical range and at the very limit of the technical sensitivity of the technique.[11]

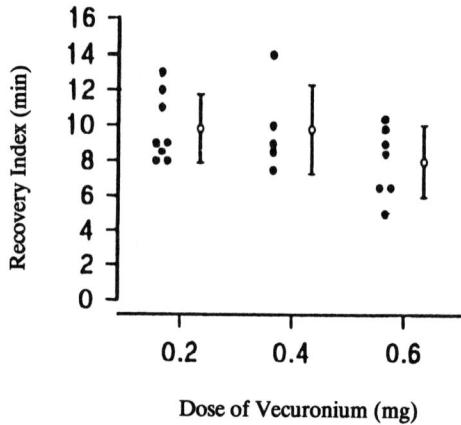

Fig. 6.11 The recovery index from three different doses of vecuronium in the isolated arm or forearm.

We have recently found the level of atracurium in plasma following release of the tourniquet in the isolated arm to be less than 10 ng/ml – a fraction of that required to produce twitch depression in the steady state (Fig. 6.9).

In an effort to test the Hull hypothesis, we used two different sets of experiments. In one set of experiments we gave 0.6 mg vecuronium to volunteers in 40 ml of saline in isolated arm experiments and measured the RI. In a further series of experiments 0.3 mg vecuronium in 20 ml of saline was given with the tourniquet on the upper forearm, or 0.2 mg vecuronium in 20 ml of saline with the tourniquet lower down the forearm. Greater than 90% block was achieved in all experiments. The RI was not significantly different, irrespective of the dose of drug used (Fig. 6.11). Thus, a threefold decrease in drug, and presumably a similar decrease in plasma concentration on release of the tourniquet, did not affect the rate of recovery of vecuronium neuromuscular block.[22]

In the other set of experiments, isolated forearm experiments were carried out on volunteers using 0.3 mg vecuronium. Following release of the tourniquet a similar dose of vecuronium was injected intravenously either at 10% recovery or at 50% recovery. If Hull's hypothesis was correct, then a sudden increase in plasma drug concentration similar to the maximum effect that could come from drug released into the circulation on deflation of the tourniquet, should have caused prolongation of the RI. No prolongation was observed[23] (Fig. 6.12).

These two sets of experiments make it unlikely that the plasma concentration of drug produced following release of the tourniquet is the cause of the slow recovery of neuromuscular block in the isolated arm experiment. These results are in accord with the results of our pharmacokinetic studies recently carried out in the isolated forearm (Fig. 6.9).

Isolated forearm and onset time

Hood et al.[24] demonstrated that, following administration of a non-depolarizing drug (atracurium and vecuronium) in the isolated forearm,

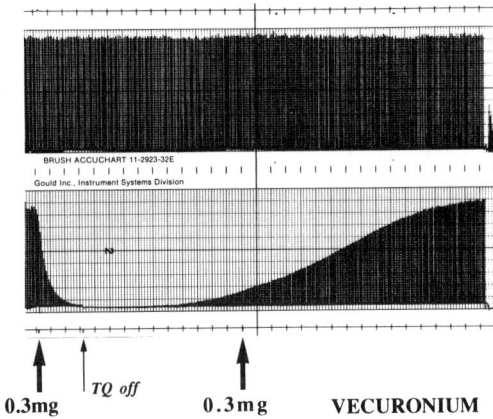

Fig. 6.12 Once the tourniquet (TQ) was released, repeated doses of 0.3 mg vecuronium did not affect the recovery index of vecuronium. Upper trace from contralateral hand.

the tourniquet could be released at 20–50% block and, in spite of an immediate loss of the driving retrograde venous pressure and the consequent reversal of the concentration gradient between synapse and extracellular fluid, the block continued to increase over the next 3–4 min (Fig. 6.13). By this means, over 95% block could usually be achieved in the absence of a continued pressure and concentration gradient. This was in marked contrast to the effect seen when C_{10} was used. Using a depolarizing drug, there was no further increase in block once the tourniquet was released. This strongly suggested that the increase in block observed with non-depolarizing drugs, but not C_{10}, was due to pharmacodynamic effects – it represented the essential onset time of non-depolarizing block in the absence of a concentration gradient for drug between extracellular fluid to the synapse. By releasing the tourniquet at 20% onset of block and measuring the time from 30 to 80% block. Feldman et al.[25]

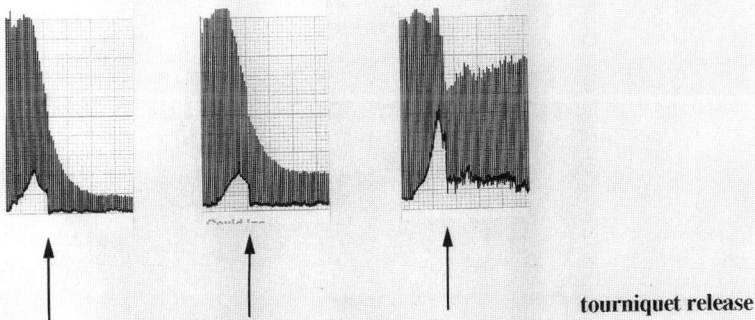

Fig. 6.13 Letting down the tourniquet at 50% onset of block is followed by an increase in atracurium and vecuronium block, but not C_{10} block.

were able to compare the onset times of vecuronium, atracurium, pancuronium and doxacurium. They found a correlation between the onset time and the RI in the isolated arm (Fig. 6.14). Thus, doxacurium had the longest onset time but also the greatest RI. England et al.[26] confirmed this relationship for pipecuronium, but found that rocuronium proved to

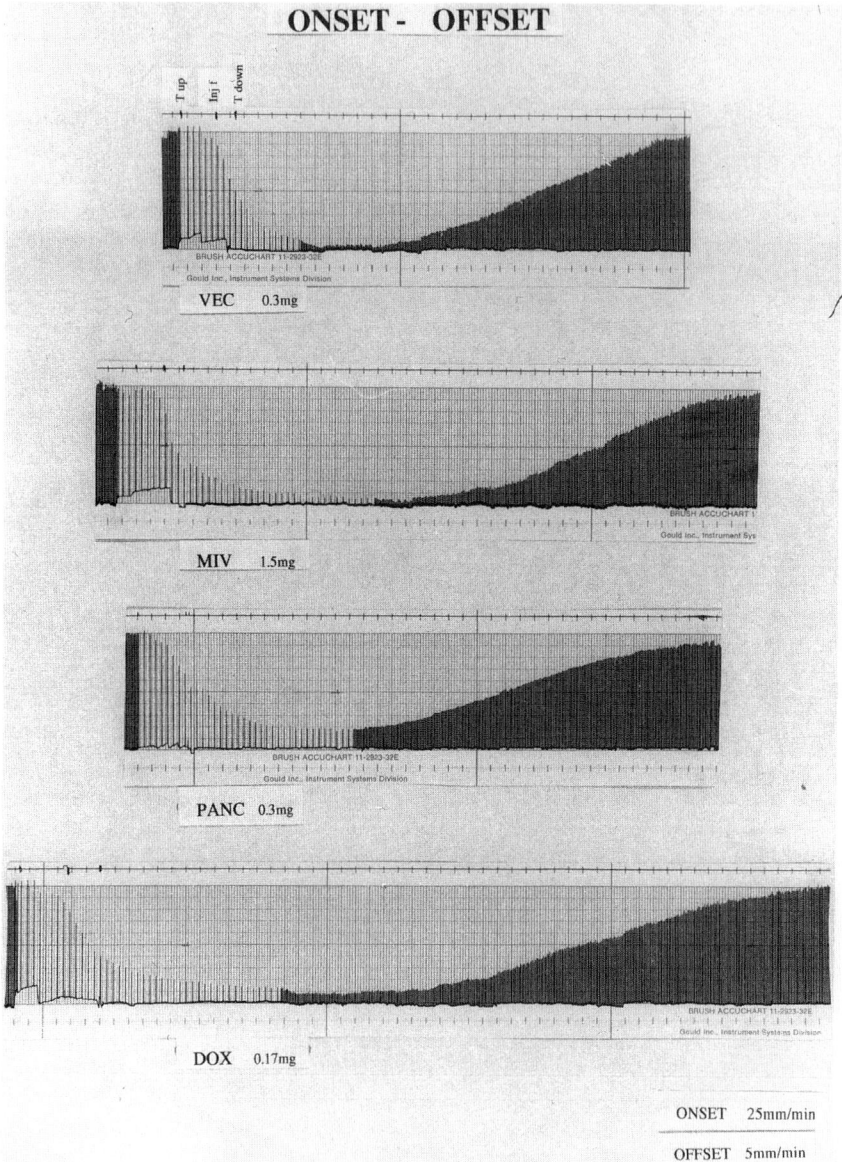

Fig. 6.14 The relation of onset of block in the isolated forearm to offset of four non-depolarizing drugs – vecuronium (VEC), atracurium (MIV), pancuronium (PANC) and doxacurium (DOX). The onset time was measured after release of the tourniquet at 20% block.

be an exception. The onset of rocuronium block was too rapid or its offset too slow to fit the general pattern observed.

Conclusion

The isolated arm experiments produce the same neuromuscular block as that found in clinical practice following a modest (ED_{95}) bolus of drug, but without the background of drug circulating in the plasma. The onset occurs due to the establishment of a pressure and concentration gradient driving fluid containing the drug into the neuromuscular synapse. Recovery occurs due to the production of a sudden high concentration gradient for the drug, encouraging a maximum rate of diffusion of free drug from the neuromuscular junction. Delay in recovery and the occurrence of different RIs for different drugs indicate that some process occurs which interferes with this washout. The observation that different drugs have differing RIs and that this depends upon the physicochemical structure of the drug implies different affinities of the drugs with the binding site. The binding process has a finite, saturable capacity. The fastest rate of recovery – that of C_{10} – is between 2.5 and 4.0 min, indicating a possible minimum washout delay. Any explanation of the recovery of neuromuscular block that does not explain these observations must be suspect. As Karl Popper has pointed out, scientific advancement occurs by disproof of existing concepts. In this instance, observations in the isolated arm more closely replicate clinical use and are far better controlled than experiments carried out in a water bath, or iontophoretic application of drug to animal muscle tissue, or the use of highly contrived techniques on isolated receptors. They must, therefore, be incorporated into any theory or model of neuromuscular block and only then should one look to the more complex experiments in animal models to test and validate these observations.

References

1. Tyrrell MF. The measurement of the force of thumb adduction. *Anaesthesia* 1969; **24:** 626
2. Feldman SA & Tyrrell MF. A new theory of the termination of action of the muscle relaxants. *Proc R Soc Med* 1970; **63:** 692–695
3. Torda T & Klonymus DH. Regional neuromuscular block. *Acta Anaesthesiol Scand* 1966; **24** (suppl): 177
4. Foldes FF. (1974) Regional intravenous neuromuscular block: a new diagnostic and experimental tool. In: *Proceedings of the 4th World Congress of Anaesthesiology.* Holland: Excerpta Medica, p. 425
5. Feldman SA, Fauvel NJ & Hood JR. Recovery from pancuronium and vecuronium administered simultaneously in the isolated forearm and the effect on recovery following administration after cross-over of drugs. *Anesth Analg* 1993; **76:** 92–95
6. Sheiner LB, Stanski DR, Vozeh S *et al.* Simultaneous modelling of pharmacokinetics and pharmacodynamics. *Clin Pharmacol Ther* 1979; **25:** 358–371
7. Stanski DR. Partition co-efficient vs dissociation rate constant as determinant of duration of neuromuscular block. *Anesthesiology* 1981; **54:** 351
8. Stanski DR & Sheiner LB. Pharmacokinetics and dynamics of muscle relaxants. *Anesthesiology* 1979; **51:** 103–105

9. Feldman SA. Affinity concept and the action of muscle relaxants. *Acts Anaesthesiol Belg* 1976; **27**: 86–96

10. Campkin NTA & Hood JR. The isolated arm. *Anaesth Pharmacol Rev* 1993; **1**: 77–80

11. Agoston S, Feldman SA & Miller RD. Plasma pancuronium concentrations and the depression of twitch height in the isolated arm following bolus injection and continuous infusion. *Anaesthesiology* 1979; **51**: 119–123

12. Pittenger CB, Morris LE & Cullen SC. Plasma estimation of *d*-tubocurarine chloride. *J Lab Clin Med* 1951; **38**: 397–401

13. Cohen EN, Brewer WM & Smith D. The metabolism and elimination of *d*-tubocurarine H[3]. *Anesthesiology* 1967; **28**: 540–546

14. Matteo RS, Spector B & Horrowitz PE. Relation of serum *d*-tubocurarine concentration to neuromuscular blockade in man. *Anesthesiology* 1974; **41**: 440–444

15. Waud BE. Serum *d*-tubocurarine concentration and twitch height. *Anesthesiology* 1975; **43**: 381–383

16. Hull CJ. Pharmacology of non-depolarizing neuromuscular blocking agents. *Br J Anaesth* 1982; **54**: 169–182

17. Documentation Geigy, table 1988. Publ Giegy Switzerland

18. Feldman SA, Soni N & Kraayenbrink MA. Effect of rate of injection on neuromuscular block produced by vecuronium. *Anesth Analg* 1989; **69**: 624–626

19. Goat VA, Feldman SA, Yeung ML *et al.* The effect of blood flow upon the activity of gallamine triethiodide. *Br J Anaesth* 1976; **48**: 69–74

20. Heneghan CPA, Findley IL, Gilbe CE & Feldman SA. Muscle blood flow and the rate of recovery from pancuronium neuromuscular block in dogs. *Br J Anaesth* 1978; **50**: 1105–1108

21. White DA & Reitan IA. Effect of blood flow in pharmacodynamics of non-depolarizing muscle relaxants using isolated limb models. *Anesthesiology* 1984; **61**: A286

22. Feldman SA. Biophase binding: its effect on recovery from non-depolarising neuromuscular block. *Anaesth Pharmacol Rev* 1993; **1**: 81–88

23. Hood JR, Campkin NTA & Feldman SA. The influence of circulating drug upon the recovery of neuromuscular block in the isolated arm. *Br J Anaesth* 1992, **69**: 226–227

24. Hood JR, Campkin NTA & Feldman SA. Depolarizing vs non-depolarizing block after early tourniquet release in the isolated forearm. *Br J Anaesth* 1993; **70**: 480

25. Feldman SA, Wu X & England AJ. Rate of onset and offset of 4 non-depolarizing neuromuscular blocking drugs. *Anaesthesia* 1995; **50**: S10–S13

26. England AJ, Redai I & Feldman SA. Rate of onset and offset of rocuronium and pipecuronium (in press)

27. Waser PG, Wiederkehr A, Chang SR & Kaiser-Schonenberger E. (1985) Kinetics and metabolism of ^{14}C labelled vecuronium in rats and mice. In: *Muscle Relaxants – Therapeutic Margins.* Agoston S, Bergmann H, Schwarz S & Steinbereithner K (eds). Vienna: W. Mandrich, pp. 15–30

7

Explanations of clinical events based on biophase binding

The acceptance of a binding compartment close to the acetylcholine receptor (AChR) which is of finite size, and for which non-depolarizing neuromuscular blocking drugs have a high affinity, makes it possible to understand many observed clinical phenomena which are otherwise difficult to explain. Although it is possible to construct models using mathematical sophistry and terms such as polyexponential effect site disposition and quasiequilibrium to try and explain these findings, a biophase binding site hypothesis allows a simple answer to many apparent paradoxes.

In the theory proposed by Feldman and colleagues,[1] it is suggested that there exists in the synaptic cleft, probably closely associated with the AChR sites, high-affinity biophase binding sites which act as the preferred acceptor for molecules of non-depolarizing drugs (Fig. 7.1). Drug occupancy of these sites deprives the AChR of ready access to the non-depolarizing agent until the binding sites are either full or else the drug dissociates from them in accordance with its K_D. Thus, onset of block will depend not upon the affinity of drug with AChR but with the biophase binding site. As the plasma level of drug falls, either due to release of the tourniquet in the isolated arm experiment or due to redistribution or

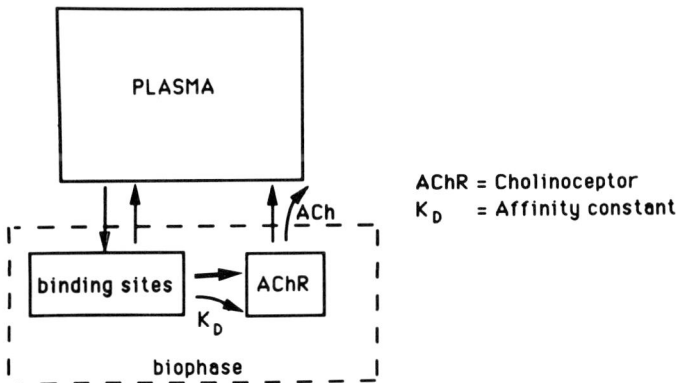

Fig. 7.1 Proposed relationship of the biophase binding sites to the acetylcholine receptor and plasma.

hydrolysis in the plasma following systemic administration, a reservoir of drug will remain in the biophase binding sites, causing a continuation of the blocking action until such time as these sites are empty. Thus the recovery of neuromuscular conduction will also be a function of the K_D of the drug.

1 Biophase binding explains why increasing blood flow, even of drug-free blood, does not cause a more rapid reversal of non-depolarizing block whereas it increases the recovery rate from decamethonium (C_{10}).
2 Biophase binding explains the priming principle, especially when a prolonged interval exists between the priming and the definitive dose of drug.
3 It offers an explanation for the slower onset of non-depolarizing block than depolarizing block and the apparent inability to produce a more rapid onset than 85–90 s unless vast doses of drug are administered.
4 It explains the relationship between onset rate, potency and offset of block.
5 It explains Armstrong and Lester's finding of increased rate of offset of tubocurare block after α cobra venom.[2] These effects, which they ascribed to buffered diffusion, cannot be explained on the basis of partitioning or blood flow.
6 It offers an explanation to the difficulty of reversing the action of non-depolarizing drugs by neostigmine when the plasma level of drug remains raised.
7 It offers an explanation of two properties of mivacurium that are otherwise difficult to understand:
   (a) Why is it possible to reverse partial block produced by mivacurium with neostigmine when its plasma clearance depends upon the presence of active plasma cholinesterase?
   (b) Why does the block produced by an ED_{95} dose of mivacurium last about 17 min when the plasma concentration falls to subclinical levels in 2–3 min? Why is its action as long as that produced by a similar dose of vecuronium, which is more slowly cleared from the plasma?

Blood flow and recovery rate

If drug were free to pass unhindered into and out from the synaptic cleft, the concentration in the region of the AChR and hence the degree of block should parallel the concentration of drug in the blood and the onset and offset of block should depend upon the concentration gradient between the synaptic cleft and the blood and blood flow. This relationship is found for onset time and blood flow (up to a limit of approximately 90 s)[3,4] with non-depolarizing drugs but no correlation is found between the recovery time and blood flow (Fig. 7.2). Even perfusing the hind limb of animals with drug-free blood and hence obtaining the maximum concentration gradient reveals no correlation between blood flow and recovery

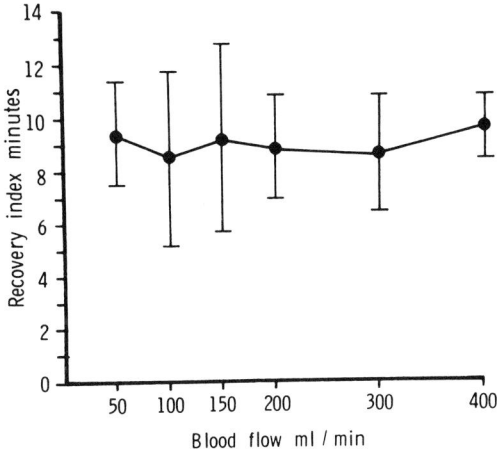

Fig. 7.2 Relationship of blood flow in the hind limb of a dog to recovery from gallamine block. From Goat et al.,[3] with permission. Increasing blood flow eight-fold does not shorten RI.

time.[6] However, when a depolarizing drug (C_{10}) is used, increasing the blood flow, even with blood-containing drug, reduces the duration of block[7] (Fig. 7.3). This strongly suggests that a mechanism exists to restrain

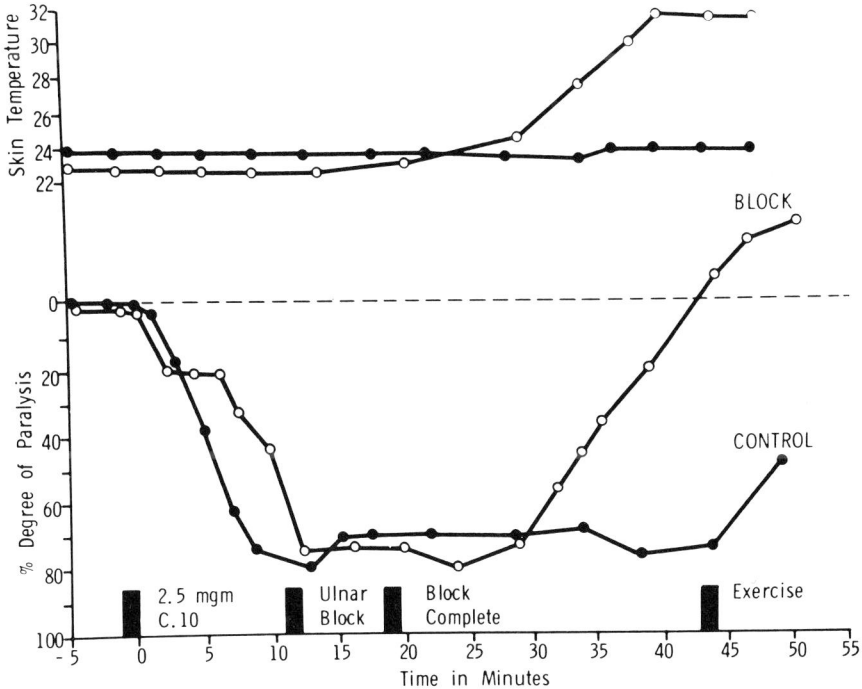

Fig. 7.3 Effect of increasing blood flow upon the rate of recovery of decamethonium. After Churchill Davidson and Richardson.[7] Increasing blood flow speeds recovery.

the easy egress of non-depolarizing drug molecules, but not depolarizing ones, from the synaptic cleft.

Priming

It has been demonstrated that the effect of priming is not diminished by a delay of up to 10 min before the definitive bolus of drug is administered.[8] It is inconceivable that the drug concentration at the receptor would remain unchanged during this time unless some mechanism exists to bind it at that site[9] (see Chapter 13).

Onset of block (Chapter 9)

The slow onset of non-depolarizing drugs compared to depolarizing ones suggests that the type of block limits the onset time. Increasing blood flow, dose and reducing potency all affect onset time but all these effects tend to reach a minimum of 90 s onset delay.[2] There is ample evidence that the drug is in the synaptic cleft before this minimum delay time but that it does not cause a postsynaptic receptor block.[10,11] It is suggested that this is because the high affinity of these drugs with biophase binding sites results in the preferential filling of these sites from which the drug is only available to the AChR at a rate determined by its dissociation constant with the biophase binding sites.

Relationship between onset time, offset time and potency

Because the speed of onset of block will be determined by the rate at which drug leaves the biophase binding sites to compete with ACh at the AChR sites, recovery of normal neuromuscular function will be determined by the rate of emptying of the binding sites. In the absence of refilling from the plasma, this will depend upon the dissociation rate constant of the drug from the biophase sites. As a result both onset and offset should be controlled by the same K_D.[12] This would not necessarily be so if onset and offset were functions of concentration gradients and blood flow alone. It remains to explain why rocuronium does not obey this condition and it is postulated that this is due to an additional important presynaptic action of this drug (Fig. 7.4).[13] (See Chapter 18.)

There is a general relationship between potency of a drug and onset time.[14-16] For equimolecular concentrations of competitive drugs, potency depends upon affinity with the receptor; the most potent drug has the greatest affinity (see p. 35). It is reasonable to suppose that if the rate-limiting step in receptor occupancy is the rate at which the drug becomes available, then potency will also be related to this function and hence to the rate of dissociation from the biophase binding sites. Hence the rate of onset, offset and potency may all have a common underlying mechanism.

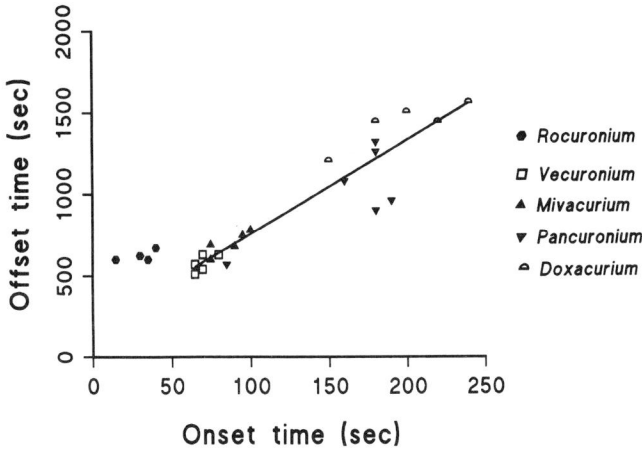

Fig. 7.4 Relationship between onset and offset times of five neuromuscular blocking drugs. Note that rocuronium does not fit the general pattern.

Buffered diffusion or physicochemical binding

The concept of buffered diffusion would explain the finding that onset of neuromuscular block by tubocurare is about 10 times faster than offset. Armstrong and Lester[2] used iontophoretically pulsed tubocurare and ACh to study this relationship. They found a ratio of onset to offset time very similar to that observed in the isolated arm, although on a very different time scale (Fig. 7.5). However, buffered diffusion does not explain why the ratio for the time from onset to offset for C_{10} is far less than that of non-depolarizing drugs in the isolated arm. Biophase binding would equally well explain the reduction in the recovery time observed by Armstrong and Lester following pretreatment with α-cobra venom and proposed as evidence for buffered diffusion. Indeed, in the rat phrenic nerve diaphragm, both onset and offset times are reduced by pretreatment with α-bungarotoxin.

The studies of Lawmin et al.[17] on the effect of hypothermia on the onset and offset of block by non-depolarizing block produced by iontophoresis in the frog demonstrated a temperature coefficient (Q_{10}) of 1.3, which is compatible with a physical process such as buffered diffusion. However, our results in the rat phrenic nerve diaphragm[18] and in humans suggest a Q_{10} of 2.4–3.0 for offset of block.[19] This high Q_{10}, which is not found for depolarizing drugs, strongly indicates that recovery from neuromuscular block in homothermic animals is related to a process involving a change in entropy, such as binding and dissociation of drug from a receptor site (see Chapter 15).

Inability to reverse non-depolarizing block

It is impossible to explain the inability of neostigmine to reverse residual curarization in the presence of a modest but significant plasma level of

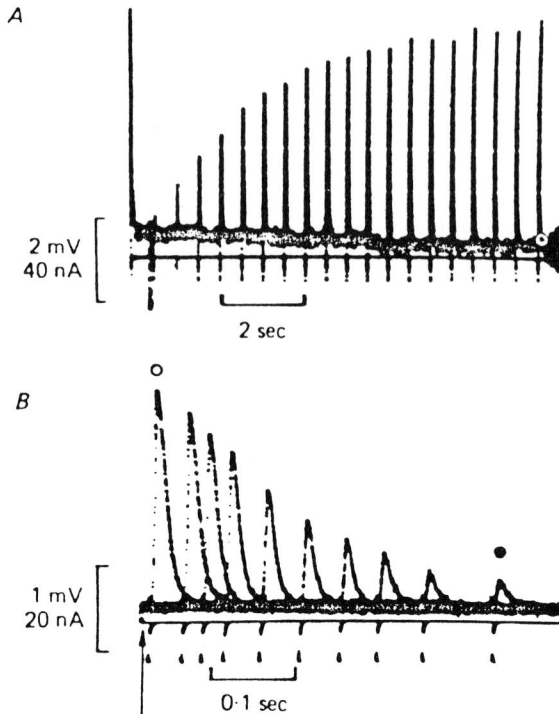

Fig. 7.5 Onset of iontophoretically induced curare block and offset induced by acetylcholine. Note that onset is approximately 20 times as quick as offset in this experiment reported by Armstrong and Lester.[2]

drug without invoking an additional mechanism in addition to simple competition at the receptor. This phenomenon was relatively common following gallamine,[20] tubocurare[21] and pancuronium.[22] On the basis of the competition theory, increasing the available ACh in the synaptic cleft by inhibiting its hydrolysis should always reverse residual block. The ability to reverse the residual block once the plasma level of drug is reduced by haemodialysis suggests that it is not due to the lack of effect of the neostigmine but to the plasma concentration of drug. This can be explained on the basis of biophase binding. A residual plasma concentration of drug would constantly refill the biophase reservoir, frustrating any effect of the raised ACh concentration produced by the neostigmine to reduce its effect at the AChR.

Mivacurium plasma clearance/duration of action paradox

In order to explain the two paradoxes observed with mivacurium – the ability to reverse its action with neostigmine and the similar duration of block with mivacurium and vecuronium following an ED_{95} dose – it is essential to accept that the neuromuscular blocking action of mivacurium outlasts the fall in its plasma concentration. During this time its action can be rapidly reversed by anticholinesterase drugs, which suggests that it produces its block by competition with ACh. However, its plasma concentration at the time of reversal must be below that required to effect a neuromuscular block and hence its half-life is not affected by the neostigmine. This can only be explained by some mechanism keeping the drug at the receptor site up to 15 min after its plasma and extracellular fluid level are reduced to subclinical levels.

In the isolated arm mivacurium block tends to be of slightly shorter duration than vecuronium, although in our series this did not reach the level of statistical significance. Following bolus injection of an ED95 dose of mivacurium, the maximum block to 75% recovery time is about 15 min,[24] whereas it is 16.0 min[25] for vecuronium (Fig. 7.6). Following 2 × ED95 dose the 0–75% recovery time for mivacurium is 16 min for mivacurium and 21 min for vecuronium.

The similarity in the rate of recovery from mivacurium and vecuronium neuromuscular block in the isolated arm and following an ED95 dose is difficult to reconcile with the very different plasma half-life of the two drugs. Using a dose of 2 × ED95 of both drugs, however, recovery from mivacurium block is significantly more rapid than after vecuronium block. This effect could be explained if the recovery from the ED95 dose of mivacurium occurred during the rapid redistribution phase of the drug. However, all the evidence points to the conclusion that recovery of neuromuscular conduction occurs long after this phase is substantially completed. Using a bioassay technique to obviate the problems of the different pharmacokinetic and potency profiles of the isomers of mivacurium, Hood[23] demonstrated the absence of a blocking concentration of mivacurium in the plasma 200 s after injecting an ED95 dose. At this time the plasma concentration of vecuronium was capable of producing about 80% block (Fig. 7.7).

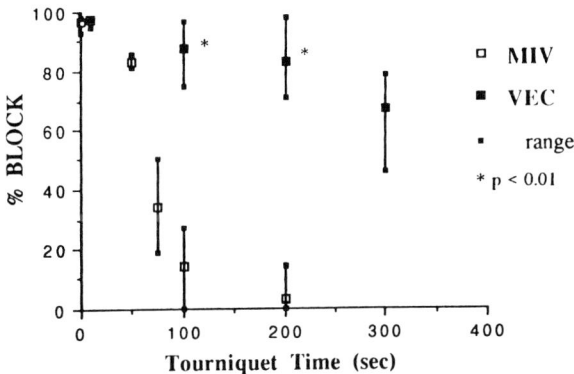

Fig. 7.6 Bioassay of the effective plasma concentration of vecuronium (VEC) and mivacurium (MIV) with time. The assay was accomplished by excluding one arm from the effect of circulating drug by means of a tourniquet. The tourniquet was released at 50 s to 50 s and the effect of the concentration of drug in the blood at that time was measured. (From Hood *et al.*,[23] with permission.)

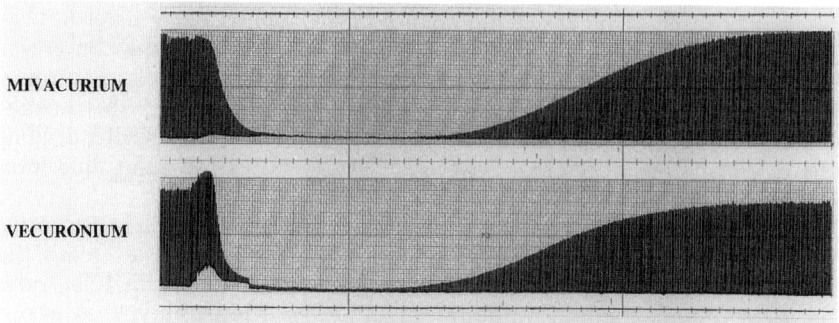

Fig. 7.7 Duration of action of mivacurium and vecuronium following an ED$_{95}$ dose of both drugs.

The impossibility of correlating the similar duration of block following a $2 \times ED_{95}$ dose of atracurium and vecuronium with more rapid plasma clearance of atracurium has been commented upon by Bevan et al.[26] and described as a paradox by Bowman.[27] In the isolated forearm the recovery index (RI) of vecuronium is shorter than that of atracurium[28] and it has been suggested that the lower affinity of vecuronium for the binding sites is offset by the slower plasma clearance of the drug producing a lesser receptor–plasma concentration gradient, after bolus injection of vecuronium. The two counterbalancing effects would be expected to produce a similar RI for both drugs. In support of this hypothesis is the finding that $1 \times ED_{95}$ dose of vecuronium has a shorter RI than an equipotent dose of atracurium (recovery occurring largely during the redistribution phase) and that with a dose of $3 \times ED_{95}$ of both drugs, vecuronium has a longer RI.

This illustrates the important secondary effect of the plasma drug concentration upon the recovery time for a drug. In a series of experiments simultaneously carried out in the Netherlands, London and San Francisco, it was demonstrated that, following the administration of pancuronium, the RI of pancuronium was quickest in the isolated arm when the plasma pancuronium concentration was lowest. It was twice as long following systemic bolus injection and four times as long following the cessation of a continuous pancuronium infusion which was associated with the highest plasma pancuronium level during recovery from the block.[29]

The importance of using a drug or technique that produces a low plasma level at the end of an operation when reversal is required was pointed out in 1976.[30] An appreciation of the time lag between the fall in plasma level of drug and degree of block, implicit in biophase binding, gives us an understanding of why it is difficult to reverse a drug and why recovery is slow when the plasma level of the drug is high. It explains why the time taken for an equipotent dose of neostigmine to reverse 90% block is longer when adminstered to drugs with a slower plasma clearance, which would be associated with a higher plasma level of drug at, the same degree of block.

Where are the biophase binding sites?

Unfortunately, we do not know where the biophase binding sites are situated, other than autoradiographic evidence that they are situated in the synapse (see Chapter 5). Waser's studies suggested that they may be associated with cholinesterase[16] but the kinetic evidence would fit better with a domain on the receptor pentamer. The pentamer is a large structure and the binding characteristics of the ACh recognition site itself may be modified 20–100-fold depending upon the contribution from neighbouring subunits. It is possible, therefore, that the biophase binding sites may be close to the ACh recognition site. One intriguing suggestion by Bowman was that only one of the two heads of all bisquaternary compounds may act as a tethering site, whilst the other competes with ACh at the AChR site (Fig. 7.8).[31] The actual number of binding sites appears to be small and finite and it is tempting to suggest that they are the cause of the apparent excess sites for binding radiolabelled curare, over and above that required to produce neuromuscular block, demonstrated by Waser. It is possible that the extra receptor sites found by Paton and Waud,[32] and described as constituting the margin of safety of neuromuscular transmission, which have to be filled before the onset of neuromuscular block can be demonstrated are the acceptor sites for the drug which constitute biophase binding (see Chapter 12).

By accepting the hypothesis that non-active binding sites are present in the biophase or effect compartment, many clinical paradoxes can be explained. The demonstration that the affinity of drugs with these putative sites varies gives us an explanation why drugs with different chemical structures but similar physical properties have different onset and offset characteristics. It explains why Daniel Bovet's assumption that drugs with an ester bond hydrolysed in the plasma, like suxamethonium and mivacurium, do not necessarily have the transient duration of action he prophesied.[33] It provides a reason why clinical usage should aim to have a low plasma drug concentration at the end of an operation rather than

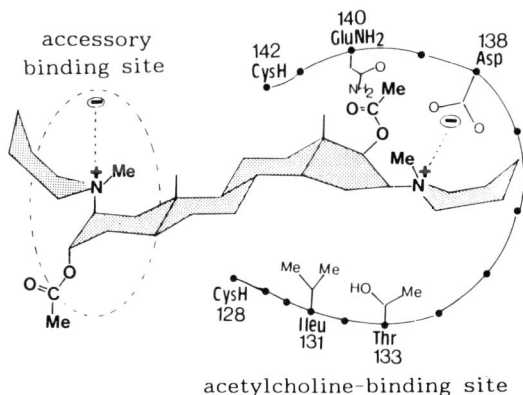

Fig. 7.8 Possible mechanism of binding of one of the two quaternary ammonium heads of a muscle relaxant whilst the other acts to compete with acetylcholine. After Bowman.[31]

rely upon the continuing action of anticholinesterase drugs in the recovery period. However, the hypothesis, although supported by overwhelming circumstantial evidence, will only be finally proven by the physical demonstration of the proposed biophase binding sites.

References

1. Feldman SA, Fauvel NJ & Hood JR. Recovery from pancuronium and vecuronium administered simultaneously in the isolated forearm and effect of recovery following adminstration after cross-over of drugs. *Anesth Analg* 1993; **76:** 92–95
2. Armstrong DL & Lester HH. The kinetics of tubocurarine action and restricted diffusion within the synaptic cleft. *J Physiol* 1979; **294:** 365–386
3. Goat V, Yeung ML, Blakeney C & Feldman SA. The effect of blood flow upon the activity of gallamine triethiodide. *Br J Anaesth* 1974; **48:** 69–72
4. Feldman SA, Soni N & Kraayenbrink MA. Effect of rate of injection on the neuromuscular block produced by vecuronium. *Br J Anaesth* 1989; **62:** 287–289
5. Henegan CPH, Findley IL, Gilbe CE & Feldman SA. Muscle blood flow and rate of recovery from pancuronium neuromuscular blockade in dogs. *Br J Anaesth* 1978; **50:** 1105–1108
6. White DA & Reitan JA. Effect of blood flow in the pharmacodynamics of non-depolarizing muscle relaxants using isolated limb model. *Anesthesiology* 1984; **61:** A286
7. Churchill Davidson HC & Richardson AT. Decamethonium iodide (C_{10}): some observations using electromyography. *Proc R Soc Med* 1952; **45:** 179–183
8. Haxby E, Hood JR, Gopinath S & Feldman SA. Mivacurium priming intervals. *Br J Anaesth* 1994; **72:** 482
9. Epstein RH & Bartkowski RR. Priming v timing: predictions of a receptor binding model of the neuromuscular junction. *Anesth Analg* 1993; **76:** 597–598
10. Feldman SA, Fauvel NJ & Harrop-Griffiths W. (1990) The onset of neuromuscular blockade. In: *Neuromuscular Blocking Agents, Past, Present and Future.* Bowman WC, Denissen PAF & Feldman SA (eds). Holland: Excerpta Medica, pp. 44–51
11. Hood JR, Campkin NTA & Feldman SA. Curare modification of suxamethonium blockade. *Anaesthesia* 1994; **49:** 682–685
12. Feldman SA, Wu X & England AJ. Rate of onset and offset of four non-depolarizing neuromuscular blocking drugs. *Anaesthesia* 1995; **50:** 510–513
13. England AJ, Redai I & Feldman SA. Ratio of onset time to recovery of pipecuronium and rocuronium. Has rocuronium a special onset mechanism? *Eur J Anaesth*, to be published
14. Bowman WC, Rodger IW, Houston J, Marshall RJ & McIndewar I. Structure action relationship amongst some desacetoxy analogues of pancuronium and vecuronium in the cat. *Anesthesiology* 1989; **69:** 57–62
15. Kopman A. Pancuronium, gallamine and *d*-tubocurarine compared. Is speed of onset inversely related to drug potency? *Anesthesiology* 1989; **70:** 915–922
16. Waser PG. (1970) On receptors in the postsynaptic membrane of the motor end plate. In: *Ciba Foundation Symposium on the Molecular Properties of Drug Receptors.* Porter R & O'Connor M (eds). London: Churchill, pp. 59–71
17. Lawmin JC, Bekavac I, Glavinovic HI, Donati F & Bevan DR. Iontophoretic study of speed of onset of various muscle relaxants. *Anesthesiology* 1992; **77:** 351–356
18. England AJ, Redai I, Richards K, Wu X & Feldman SA. The effect of hypothermia on the rate of recovery of vecuronium, atracurium and decamethonium. *Anaesthesia*, to be published
19. England AJ. Personal communication
20. Feldman SA & Levi AJ. Prolonged paresis following gallamine. *Br J Anaesth* 1963; **35:** 804–806

21. Fairley HB. Prolonged intercostal block due to a relaxant. *Br Med J* 1950; **1:** 986

22. Abrams RE & Hornbein T. Inability to reverse pancuronium blockade in a patient with renal and hepatic disease. *Anesthesiology* 1975; **42:** 362–363

23. Hood JR. A mivacurium bioassay. Presented at Anaesthetic Research Society Meeting, London 1993

24. Robertson EN, Booij JHDJ, Frogen RS & Crul JF. Clinical comparison of atracurium and vecuronium (ORG NC45). *Br J Anaesth* 1983; **54:** 125–129

25. Savarese JJ, Ali HH, Basta SJ *et al.* The clinical pharmacology of mivacurium chloride (BW B1090V). *Anesthesiology* 1988; **68:** 723–732

26. Bevan DR, Bevan JC & Donati F. (1988) Non-depolarizing relaxant. In: *Muscle Relaxants in Clinical Anesthesia.* New York: Year Book, p. 147

27. Bowman WC. (1990) Clinically used non-depolarizing neuromuscular blocking drugs. In: *Pharmacology of Neuromuscular Function.* London: Wright, p. 168

28. Lawmin JC, Hood JR, Campkin NTA & Feldman SA. Recovery of atracurium and vecuronium neuromuscular block in the isolated forearm. *Br J Anaesth* 1993; **71:** 730–731

29. Agoston S, Feldman SA & Miller RD. Plasma pancuronium concentrations and the depression of twitch height in the isolated arm, following bolus injection and continuous infusion. *Anesthesiology* 1979; **51:** 119–123

30. Feldman SA. Affinity concept of the action of the muscle relaxants. *Acta Anaesthesiol Belg* 1976; **27:** 89–91

31. Bowman WC. (1992) The discovery and evolution of aminosteroidal neuromuscular blocking agents. In: *The Development of Aminosteroid Neuromuscular Blocking Agents,* Denissen PAF (ed.) Brussels: Interface Symposium, p. 15

32. Paton WDM & Waud DR. The margin of safety of neuromuscular transmission. *J Physiol* 1967; **191:** 59–90

33. Bovet D, Bovet-Nitti F, Guarins S *et al.* Propieta farmacodenamiche di alcuni derivati della succinylcholina defati di azione curarica. *Rendic Istituto Superiore di Sanita* 1949; **12:** 106–137

8

Pharmacokinetics and pharmacokinetic models

Pharmacokinetics is the study of the uptake distribution and elimination of drugs. The study necessitates the measurement of plasma concentration of drugs against time. By studying the effect of age, disease and changes in body function on the drug concentration in the plasma during the passage of time, certain deductions can be made about the likely effect of these conditions on the action of the drug in clinical practice. In this way the characteristics of a drug may be assessed and valid assumptions can be made.

The application of pharmacokinetics to neuromuscular blocking drugs started when reliable methods of determining the plasma concentrations of these drugs became available. Although Pittinger et al.[1] described a colorimetric method of analysing tubocurare it was not easily reproducible. In the 1960s Cohen and colleagues[2] used tritiated neuromuscular blocking drugs to measure the plasma concentration of tubocurare and Feldman, working with Cohen, used the method to determine the role of the kidney in eliminating gallamine from the blood.[3] Autoradiographic studies carried out at the same time demonstrated the complex dynamics associated with the distribution of these drugs.[4] It revealed that, far from following simple physical laws, with predictable rates of mixing and equilibration in the tissues, the blocking agents studied demonstrated rapid early passage into the cells of the liver and kidney against the concentration gradient and a late redistribution to muscle water. Gallamine was rapidly concentrated in the mucopolysaccharide of cartilage in spite of its poor blood flow.[5] At about the same time, Waser[6] demonstrated the rapid concentration of toxiferine and calabash curares in the synaptic cleft. His work showed that repeated washing failed to dislodge the drug, which he believed was bound to receptor substance. Only when decamethonium was used was there any evidence of drug entering muscle cells – a finding confirmed by Creese et al.[7]

From these and other observations it was evident that the presence of variable and unpredictable active transport of these drugs, together with many binding sites of differing affinities, would make any attempt to characterize the effect of these drugs at the neuromuscular junction from their plasma concentration alone virtually impossible.

The observation by Matteo et al.[8] that, following the administration of tubocurare, the plasma level peaked and then fell whilst at the same time the neuromuscular block also peaked and then declined led to the assumption that this was a cause and effect and it was the reduction in plasma drug concentration that determined the speed of recovery from neuromuscular block. The danger of this type of assumption has been well-recognized by scientists[9] and was described at the time.[10] However, it failed to inhibit the modelling of plasma concentration against effect in a series of mathematical concepts that became increasingly separated from physiological and pharmacological reality. It was suggested that these models 'explained' or 'allowed predication' of observed events following administration of neuromuscular blocking drugs when in effect they merely rearrange observed events in a mathematical display; they remain what they are – models. Because the uptake and distribution of these drugs do not follow physical laws, the usefulness of trying to predict or explain events which are mathematically chaotic in conventional terms is limited. They are but another method of displaying numbers, like bar charts or histograms; they do not produce any new measurements and yet it is measurement that is the basis of science. Whilst they may be a useful way of comparing the behaviour of one drug with another, they have a very limited application in the study of pharmacokinetics of neuromuscular blocking drugs.

Pharmacokinetic information is useful and it can be important. The distribution volumes reflect likely drug dosages; clearance rates indicate the relative ability to reverse the action of the drug; the volume of distribution in the steady state gives information about the dosage requirements of drugs during continuous infusion, etc. Pharmacokinetics allows one drug to be compared with another. The effect of disease, age, temperature or other drugs upon these parameters may help us use these drugs safely in different circumstances. The problem lies in interpreting these results in non-equilibrium conditions in terms of the effect observed. Only when equilibrium has been established between the plasma drug concentration and the receptor producing an observed, measured effect can one have confidence in relating them as cause and effect.

References

1. Pittenger CB, Morris LE & Cullen SC. Colorimetric method for the assay of d-tubocurarine chloride. *J Lab Clin Med* 1951; **38:** 397
2. Cohen EN, Brewer WM & Smith D. The metabolism and elimination of d-tubocurarine H_3. *Anesthesiology* 1967; **28:** 540
3. Feldman SA, Cohen EN & Golling R. The excretion of H_3 gallamine in the dog. *Anesthesiology* 1969; **30:** 593
4. Cohen EN, Corbascio A & Fleisclli G. The distribution and fate of d-tubocurare. *J Pharmacol Exp Ther* 1965; **147:** 120
5. Cohen EN, Hood N & Golling R. Use of whole body autoradiography for the determination of uptake and distribution of labelled muscle relaxants in the rat. *Anesthesiology* 1968; **21:** 987
6. Waser PG. Receptor localization by autoradiographic techniques. *Ann NY Acad Sci* 1967; **144:** 737–742
7. Creese R, Taylor DB & Tilten B. Studies with muscle relaxant labelled with I^{131}. *Science* 1957; **125:** 494

8. Matteo RS, Spector S & Harrowitz PE. Relation of serum *d*-tubocurarine concentration to neuromuscular blockade in man. *Anesthesiology* 1974; **41:** 440–443

9. Huff D. (1979) *How to Lie with Statistics.* London: Pelican Books

10. Feldman SA. Serum dTc and neuromuscular blockade in man. *Anesthesiology* 1975; **42:** 644–645

Onset of action of non-depolarizing drugs

The search for a non-depolarizing neuromuscular blocking drug with a rapid onset of action has long been regarded as the last obstacle in achieving the prize of the ideal relaxant. Although few would now be as bold as I have been in the past in suggesting that achieving this aim is impossible, as yet no non-depolarizing drug acting at the postsynaptic receptor site has an onset time as short as that of the depolarizing drugs such as suxamethonium (40 s) or decamethonium (C_{10}; 60 s) when given in a dose of $2 \times ED_{95}$. New experimental agents such as ANQ9040 did approach the 60 s onset time of C_{10} but it is by no means certain that this drug, with its marked train-of-four (TOF) fade during onset, acted primarily at the postsynaptic receptor site.[1] Of all the presently available drugs, rocuronium comes nearest to this desirable characteristic. Typically with this drug, the initial rapid onset to 60–70% block is in 40–60 s; it is associated with marked tetanic fade followed by a slower final onset phase to complete the abolition of the twitch response[2] (Fig. 9.1a). This suggests that this drug also might owe its more rapid onset of action to an early presynaptic action. This is supported by the presence of marked tetanic fade following the administration of rocuronium in the rat phrenic nerve diaphragm preparation even when the dose is insufficient to cause twitch depression (Fig. 9.1b).

Why is non-depolarizing block slow in onset?

Various theories have been advanced to explain the slow onset of non-depolarizing block but to be acceptable, any hypothesis must also explain why depolarizing drugs do not share the same slow-onset characteristics. Amongst the various explanations that have been suggested are the following:

1 Blood flow.
2 Concentration gradient and dose.
3 Potency.
4 Access to receptor.
5 Biophase binding.

(a)

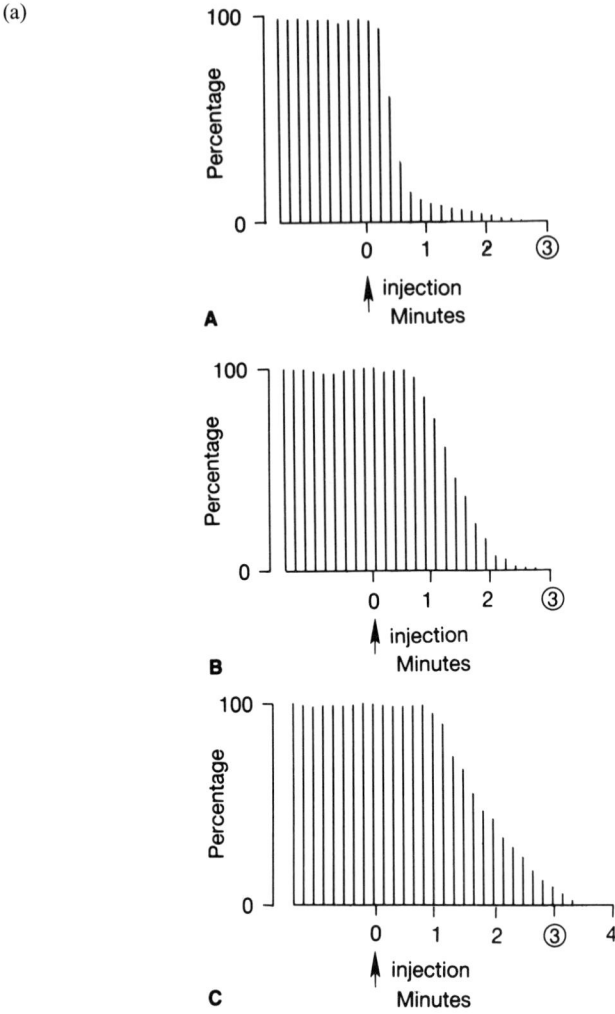

A

injection
Minutes

B

injection
Minutes

C

injection
Minutes

(b)

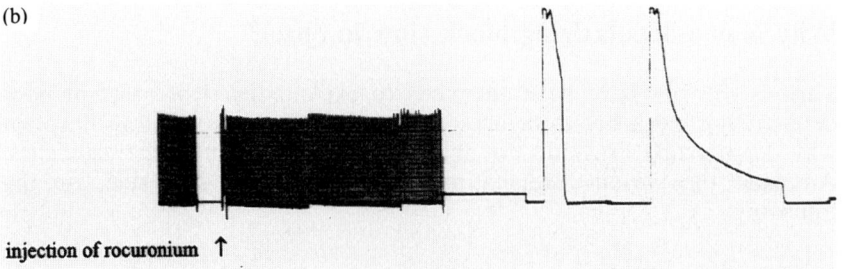

injection of rocuronium ↑

Fig. 9.1 (a) Onset of (A) rocuronium block compared to (B) vecuronoium and (C) pancuronium demonstrates rapid onset to 70–80% block. (b) The response to a 1- and 6-s 50 Hz tetanic stimulus in the isolated rat phrenic nerve diaphragm preparation after two-fifths of an ED_{50} dose of rocuronium. Small doses of rocuronium are associated with marked tetanic fade.

Blood flow

It has been suggested that the blood flow to muscle is too low to allow a rapid onset of action of non-depolarizing drugs.[3] This is clearly incorrect, as if true it would also prevent a rapid onset of depolarizing block. It fails to explain why it is possible to achieve the onset of block in 60 s with vecuronium at quite low concentrations in the water bath of the phrenic nerve diaphragm preparation of a mouse, in spite of the complete absence of any blood flow. If blood flow alone determined the distribution of drug it fails to explain why autoradiographs clearly demonstrate uptake of gallamine and aminosteroid drugs in high concentration in the cartilage of rats within 3 min of injection (Fig. 9.2) despite a poor arterial blood supply.[4] It can be readily demonstrated in patients that molecules of vecuronium and tubocurare reach the synaptic cleft as early as suxamethonium, for when they are administered together the non-depolarizing drug affects the onset of the suxamethonium block.[5] It is also possible to detect the onset of neuromuscular block with vecuronium less than 60 s after $2 \times ED_{95}$ dose by using 1 Hz rate of stimulation, yet the block with 0.1 Hz stimulation takes 3 min to occur.[6] The low blood flow of 3 ml/min per g given to support this hypothesis is one of the lowest reported and the flow in normal postural muscles at rest may exceed this figure threefold.[7] In active muscles it is always greater than the figure used in Waud's calculations. Since no non-depolarizing relaxant has been demonstrated in muscle itself in the early stages of neuromuscular block, the concept of onset being directly related to muscle blood flow has to be questioned. Indeed, the blood flow to the neuromuscular junction itself may differ from that to muscle, as muscle has a separate blood supply (see Chapter 2). The neuromuscular junction has a relatively luxurious perfusion from vessels accompanying the motor nerve.

As the neuromuscular blocking drugs are all water-soluble and rapidly distributed in the extracellular fluid (ECF), they are not dependent upon the blood supply to a particular structure or organ but produce their effect largely through diffusion from the ECF into the synaptic cleft and hence to the receptor site. Obviously the amount of drug delivered to a muscle cannot exceed the product of the plasma flow and the drug content, but the drug can be demonstrated to diffuse rapidly into the ECF,

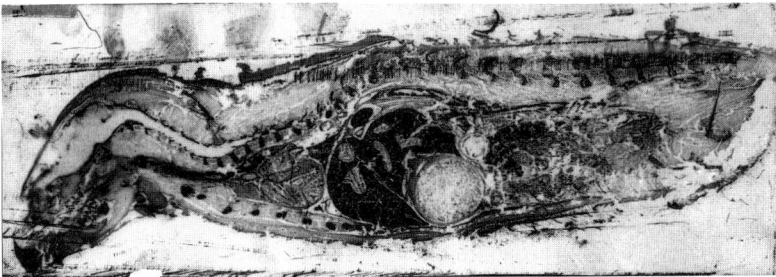

Fig. 9.2 Autoradiograph of rat sacrificed 2 min after receiving H^3 gallamine. Note the high concentration of H^3 gallamine in the cartilage.

interstitial muscle, water and into the synaptic cleft, provided a concentration gradient exists between the blood to the tissues around the muscle and the receptor.

There is a general relationship between cardiac output, blood flow and onset time. However, the relationship becomes of less consequence at the high rates of flow found in normal muscle. Thus an abnormally low cardiac output or restricted blood flow may prolong onset time but there is no reason to suppose that increasing the blood flow to muscle artificially will greatly shorten the onset time of block. This was clearly demonstrated by Goat et al.[9] using gallamine. They used a calibrated roller pump to deliver a blood flow of from 50 to 400 ml/min through the hind limb of dogs (Fig. 9.3). The more marked relationship between flow and onset time observed at low flow would fit with the concept that it was the log of the concentration of drug delivered in the blood that produced the effect on onset time. However, it is noticeable from these experiments that there is relatively little decrease in onset time once the blood flow reached 300 ml/min and that increasing the flow from 300 to 400 ml/min only results in reducing the onset time from 100 to 90 s. Even at abnormally high rates of flow, an onset time shorter than 90 s was not achieved.

The small effect of increased blood flow on onset time has been studied following unilateral sympathetic block or as a result of reactive hyperaemia, following 5 min tourniquet ischaemia, which increases blood flow 10-fold.[7] In neither circumstance was the onset of block in the arm with increased blood more than 10% quicker than in the control arm. However, increasing the stimulation rate 10-fold did appear to induce a more rapid onset of vecuronium block and some of this effect may be due to an increase in blood flow consequent upon the increased muscle activity caused by the faster rate of stimulation.

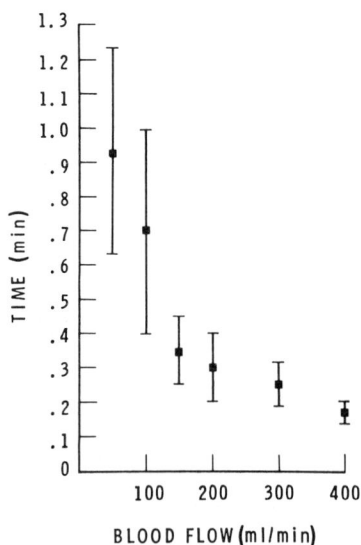

Fig. 9.3 Relationship between blood flow and onset of gallamine block in the hind leg of a dog. Note that the effect is most marked at low blood flows. Goat et al.,[9] with permission.

The effect of a low cardiac output, like low blood flow, is to reduce the rate of onset of block of both non-depolarizing and depolarizing drugs (Fig. 9.4). Once very low blood flows are produced then an element of hypoxia occurs which affects the onset of block and considerably prolongs the duration of any type of neuromuscular block. Few anaesthetists have not waited expectantly for the delayed onset of fasciculations heralding the arrival of suxamethonium at the neuromuscular junction of elderly patients with poor cardiac output. A similar condition was simulated by Feldman et al.[10] by administering vecuronium in a slow infusion over 5 min. They found an approximate doubling of the time to the onset of maximum block due to the slow injection of drug. However, even this fails to compensate at very low concentrations.

If a drug is administered by close intra-arterial injection, the effect on blood flow is minimized. Yet, in spite of this, the onset time of intra-arterial vecuronium and tubocurare has been found to be 2–3 min in animals. As the blood flow is the vehicle delivering the drug to the muscle and the neuromuscular synapse, low flow can be compensated for by increasing the plasma drug content. Thus the effect of a low blood flow or a low cardiac output on onset can be offset, to some extent, by increasing the dose of drug.

It is evident that in normal circumstances blood flow cannot explain the slower onset of non-depolarizing drugs compared to depolarizing agents. Only in conditions of seriously reduced blood flow or low plasma drug concentration does blood flow appear significantly to limit the rate of onset of block. However, even this fails to compensate at very low concentrations.

Concentration of drug in the blood

Theoretically, the onset of block produced by receptor occupancy should relate to the log of the number of molecules of drug to which the acetyl-

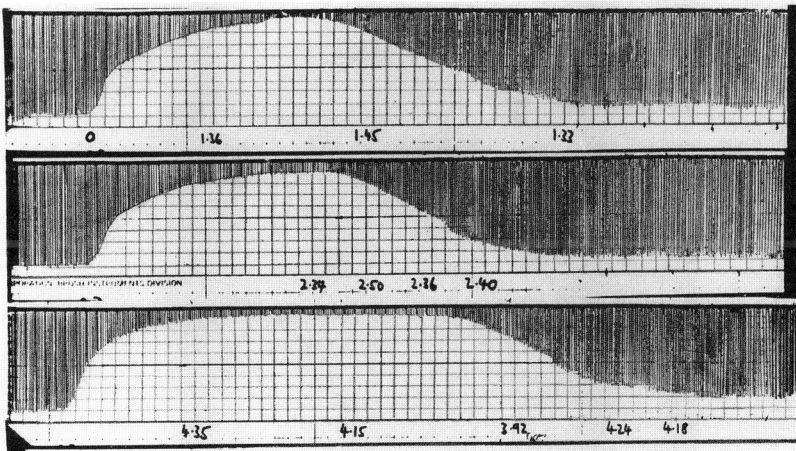

Fig. 9.4 Effect of low cardiac output on onset of pancuronium block in dogs. The fall in cardiac output was produced by inflating a balloon in the atrium of the heart. Top trace cardiac output average 1.36 l/min during onset; lower trace 4.35 l/min.

choline receptor (AChR) is exposed. A log dose relationship with onset time can generally be demonstrated. However, as the dose is increased the relationship is lost and a time barrier revealing a minimum onset time of 90–100 s is found. This has been studied in most detail with vecuronium as this is the one drug that is so lacking in side-effects that multiples of the ED_{95} up to $10 \times ED_{95}$ can be safely administered to patients. Figure 9.5 illustrates the effect on the onset time of various doses of vecuronium recorded by different authors using a variety of techniques. It is remarkable that in spite of lack of control of the protocols used the results are remarkably consistent. Interestingly, the 90 s minimum onset time demonstrated is similar to the minimum onset time achieved when the blood flow was increased to 400 ml/min in the dog in the experiments of Goat et al.[9] using gallamine.

The problem of how to explain the rapid onset of depolarizing drugs such as suxamethonium and C_{10} remains. It has been suggested that because of the rapid metabolism of suxamethonium in the plasma, a relative excess of drug molecules is administered, establishing a highly favourable concentration gradient between the ECF and the synaptic cleft and minimizing the inevitable delay caused by drug passing into a large diluting volume.[8] However, mivacurium, which is hydrolysed in a similar manner to suxamethonium and at a rate that is approximately 80% as fast, has an even slower onset in $2 \times ED_{95}$ dose than vecuronium. This hypothesis also fails to explain why C_{10}, which is not hydrolysed in plasma and should therefore not have the same favourable ECF–synaptic cleft gradient as suxamethonium, has a more rapid onset time than non-depolarizing drugs.

If one calculates the number of drug molecules administered in equipotent doses of C_{10}, vecuronium, atracurium and tubocurare, they are all of a similar order.[6] Of the non-depolarizing drugs in common use,

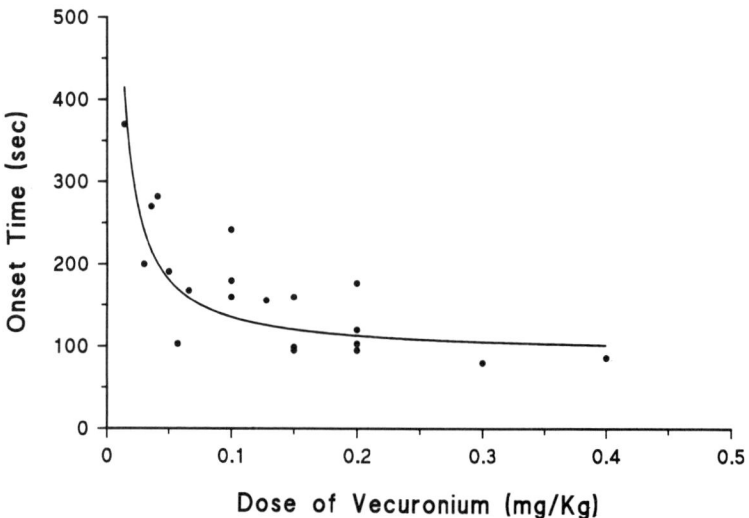

Fig. 9.5 Relationship between the dose of vecuronium and onset time of block.

atracurium requires a greater number of molecules to produce 95% block than all the others except for gallamine. Gallamine requires a considerably higher concentration of drug to effect a block; however, in clinical practice gallamine has only a marginally more rapid onset time than tubocurare; atracurium is slower in onset than vecuronium and all are appreciably slower in onset than C_{10}.

Thus, although it appears possible to increase the rate of onset to maximum block by increasing the dose of drug, there is a limit to this effect within the clinical range. A similar effect was reported by Healy et al.[11] They demonstrated that increasing the dose of both atracurium and vecuronium increased the rate of onset but this effect reached an asymptote at 100–120 s (Fig. 9.6). It is possible to produce a faster onset of neuromuscular block when $20 \times ED_{95}$ and higher doses are administered in experiments in animals. However, in the doses used in humans there is little evidence that the faster onset of the depolarizing drug C_{10} and suxamethonium relative to the non-depolarizing drugs is due to a greater number of drug molecules administered or to the rapid hydrolysis of suxamethonium.

Potency

In 1966 Waser[12] produced evidence, that with the exception of tubocurare, all the calabash curare preparations he studied demonstrated a relationship between potency, rate of onset of block and recovery rate (Fig. 9.7). The more potent the drug, the slower the rate of onset, the longer the duration of action and the slower the rate of recovery. The potency of a drug is related to the affinity of the drug with the receptor. Thus, drugs of high affinity are more potent, whereas drugs bound with less avidity,

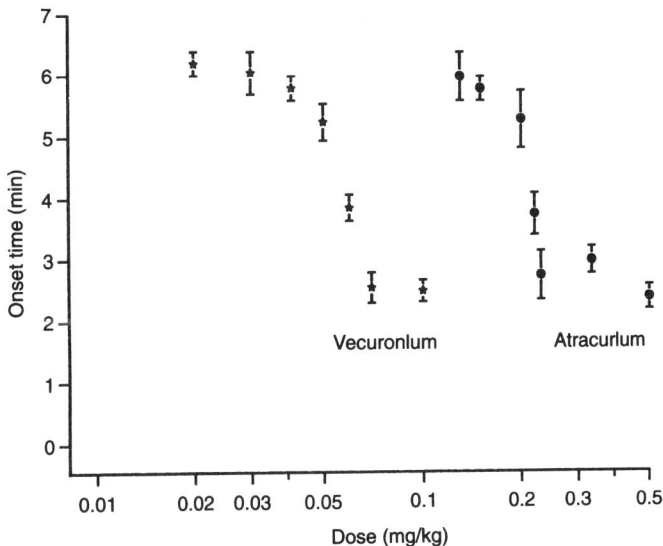

Fig. 9.6 Relationship between dose of atracurium and vecuronium and onset of block. From Healy et al.,[11] with permission.

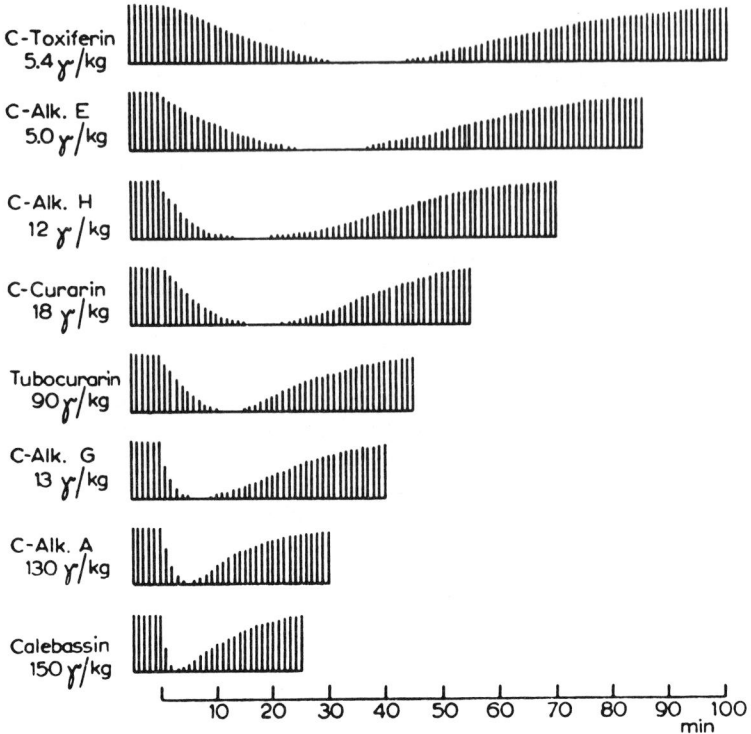

Fig. 9.7 Relationship between onset time and potency of calabash curares. Note tubocurare is an exception. From Waser,[12] with permission.

which rapidly associate and dissociate from the receptor, are less potent. The problem left unanswered is, on to what do these agents become bound? Waser[13] believed that they were bound to the receptor, or if not the AChR itself, then possibly to cholinesterase, closely associated with the receptor. The presence of drug apparently bound at the receptor areas was demonstrated in many of his early elegant autoradiographs using a variety of drugs (see Chapter 5).

The relationship between potency and onset time of three non-depolarizing drugs was meticulously mapped by Kopman.[14] In a study in patients he produced evidence that supported the concept that low potency of a non-depolarizing agent was associated with more rapid onset irrespective of the chemical grouping of the agent used. In a series of experiments in which various non-depolarizing drugs were introduced into the synapse of frogs using an iontophoretic micropipette technique, Lawmin et al.[15] found a similar relationship. They found that the more potent drugs with the lowest dissociation constants had the slowest onset and offset time in the frog. However, this technique does not allow the actual dose of drug administered to be accurately controlled and the frog neuromuscular junction is not necessarily a good model for humans.

Bowman *et al.*[16] studied the relationship of potency and onset time in the aminosteroid series of drugs and again confirmed the relationship between potency and onset time (Fig. 9.8). However, they demonstrated that, even with the least potent agent – one that was so weak that it required constant injection to produce a block – the onset time to maximum block was not reduced below 90 s, i.e. longer than the slowest depolarizing drug, C_{10}. It is of interest that once again the fastest onset time that could be produced was 90 s. This is the same as the fastest onset time produced by increasing the dose of vecuronium to $10 \times ED_{95}$ and the same minimum onset delay observed using gallamine when the blood flow to the hind limb of a dog was increased maximally.

In our own experiments in the isolated forearm we have found that there is a relationship between the speed of onset and rate of recovery.[18] Thus one can grade the relaxants studied from vecuronium, atracurium, pancuronium, pipecuronium to doxacurium. However, there appears to be one exception to this relationship – rocuronium.[19] Rocuronium has a faster onset time in the isolated forearm and in patients than does vecuronium but both drugs have a recovery index of a similar order.

Kim *et al.*[17] investigated the paradoxical observation that, following a bolus ED_{95} dose of mivacurium or atracurium, mivacurium, the more

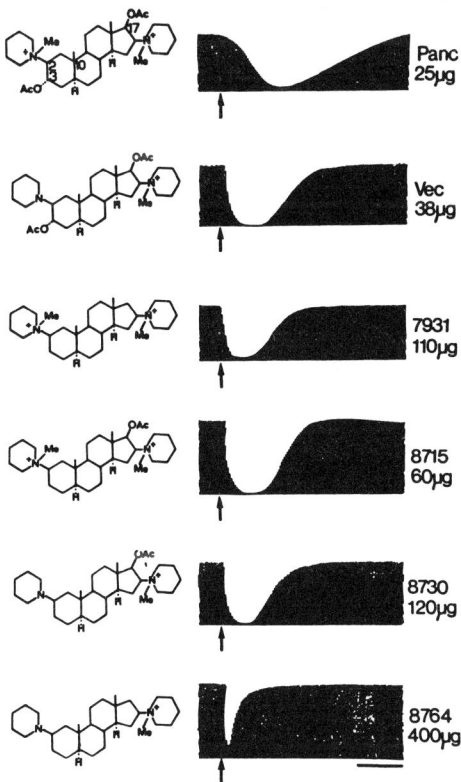

Fig. 9.8 Relationship between onset of block and potency of aminosteroid relaxants. After Bowman *et al.*[16]

potent drug, has the shorter recovery time. Using mivacurium in one isolated forearm and atracurium in the other they demonstrated that by eliminating the effect of drug in the plasma the recovery of mivacurium, the more potent drug, was longer than that of atracurium. They concluded that the apparent paradox appears to be due to the slower plasma clearance of atracurium.

In order to study onset time in the isolated forearm the tourniquet is released as the block is starting to develop. By releasing the tourniquet at 20% block and allowing the block to develop to 80%, the 25–75% onset time can be determined whilst it is only minimally influenced by the concentration of drug in the blood and not affected by the venous backpressure. It is of interest that if C_{10} is used there is no further progression of block once the tourniquet is released. Rocuronium consistently demonstrates less increase in block than vecuronium, atracurium or doxacurium when the tourniquet is released. Indeed, its onset profile in the isolated arm is between that of vecuronium and C_{10}.

These experiments demonstrate that whatever is responsible for the slower onset of the non-depolarizing drugs is associated with establishing a reservoir of drug in the synapse that allows an increase in block once the plasma concentration falls and that this does not occur with C_{10}. The fact that non-depolarizing block increases from 20% to 75–90% following the release of the tourniquet and in spite of the fall in plasma concentration of drug demonstrates that the drug molecules required for this effect are already in the biophase at the moment when the tourniquet is deflated, even though this may be only 10 s after injection of the drug. These findings, together with the observed evidence that vecuronium and tubocurare can gain access to the synapse in the time it takes for suxamethonium to start to produce its block, strongly support the view that the drug reaches the biophase rapidly but that it takes a finite time to achieve an adequate concentration at the AChR to produce block and it is this delay that largely contributes to the slow onset.

The time taken for onset to occur once the drug is in the biophase varies from drug to drug and appears to correlate with the time taken for the recovery of the block. Thus it is generally shorter for drugs with rapid recovery. Once biophase occupancy has occurred it does not require a continuing concentration gradient of drug, from the plasma to the biophase, to produce the AChR occupancy necessary for the onset of neuromuscular block, although if such a gradient is present it appears to reduce the onset time marginally.

In general, there exists a relationship between onset time and drug potency (affinity) and offset time for non-depolarizing drugs. Certain exceptions occur. Rocuronium is more rapid in onset than would be predicted from its offset (or its offset is slower than would be predicted from its potency).[19] Atracurium is less potent than vecuronium but has a similar onset and recovery profile in doses of $2 \times ED_{95}$.

Penetration of the synapse

It has been suggested that the slower onset of the non-depolarizing relaxant drugs compared to depolarizing agents is due to their molecular bulk. It is suggested that the bulky pachycurares, such as tubocurare, would require a greater time to penetrate the Schwann cell membrane than the slim, linear leptocurares such as C_{10} or suxamethonium. This explanation is unlikely. It can be demonstrated in the isolated forearm that even if the tourniquet is deflated when only 20% block has been achieved some 10–20 s after completion of injection, the block continues to develop and 80–90% block is eventually achieved. Obviously drug in sufficient quantity to produce 80–90% AChR occupancy eventually must have been present in the synapse when the tourniquet was released. It is unlikely that the Schwann cell membrane imposes any barrier to the ingress or egress of water-soluble molecules, even those of a greater size than the pachycurares.

In a series of experiments that conclusively confirm the early presence of vecuronium and tubocurare in the biophase, Feldman et al.[5] demonstrated that if vecuronium is given together with suxamethonium, or tubocurare is administered 10 s before suxamethonium,[20] then the antagonist drug reaches the biophase sufficiently rapidly to affect the subsequent

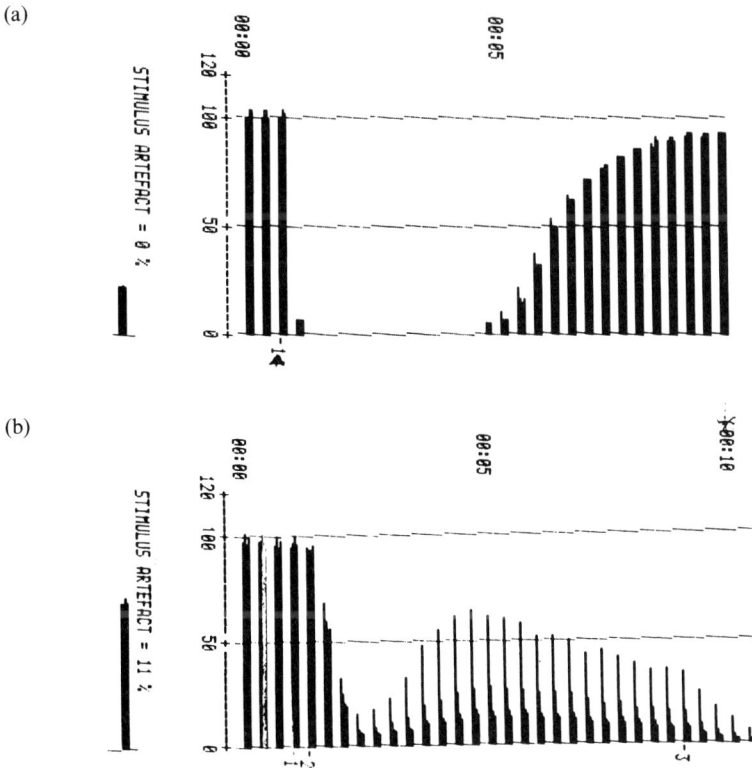

Fig. 9.9 Relaxograph train-of-four trace. (a) 1 = Suxamethonium 1 mg/kg; (b) 1 = Tubocurare 0.125 mg/kg; 2 = suxamethonium 1 mg/kg. Note that prior administration of a small dose of tubocurare affects the onset of suxamethonium block and modifies the extent of the block. It confirms that molecules of tubocurare are present in the synapse during onset of suxamethonium block.

depolarizing block produced by the suxamethonium (Fig. 9.9). In order for the vecuronium or tubocurare to affect the rate and degree of the suxamethonium block, molecules of antagonist drug must be present in the synaptic cleft when the agonist block was occurring, i.e. within the time scale of the start of the onset of the suxamethonium block.

It is therefore unlikely that it is the difficulty of non-depolarizing drug reaching the synaptic cleft that is the cause of the difference in the onset time of depolarizing and non-depolarizing agents.

Biophase binding

What then is the cause of the slow onset of non-depolarizing drugs? Feldman et al.[5] suggested that the cause might be the need for the non-depolarizing drugs to occupy a greater proportion of the AChR pool than non-depolarizing drugs before their effect became manifest. According to the margin of safety concept, depolarizing block would occur if about 20% of the receptors were affected by the drug. However, a non-depolarizing drug would have to occupy 80% or more of the receptors before depression of twitch response was produced. The Hill equation and the log-dose effect suggest that relatively few drug molecules are required to occupy the initial 20% of the receptors compared to the number required to occupy 80%. This theory is superficially attractive but it fails to explain why even when large doses of drug are administered or a drug of very low affinity used, a 90 s delay in onset occurs. It would be expected that giving a large dose, i.e. $10 \times ED_{95}$ of vecuronium, would produce an overwhelming number of drug molecules and that the onset delay would have been reduced at least to the same level as that for suxamethonium block.

In order to explain all the observations, we have proposed that following the intravenous administration of a non-depolarizing drug it is rapidly taken up by high-affinity sites in the biophase. These sites act like a sponge which retains water after it has been removed from the bath; thus, as the plasma level of drug falls rapidly following injection, the biophase retains drug molecules. The drug will leave these binding sites in accordance with its particular affinity. Weak drugs with low affinity will leave more rapidly than more potent high-affinity ones. Once free of these binding sites, drug may either pass out into the synaptic cleft and plasma or on to the AChR. The greater the residual plasma concentration of drug, the more likely are molecules that have dissociated from the binding sites to react with the AChR and produce block. Only if very large doses of drug are administered will the binding capacity of the biophase be overwhelmed. Evidence from isolated forearm experiments suggests that this occurs at high drug concentrations as these binding sites have a finite capacity. Some concept of the size of this binding compartment can be deduced from the effect of the dose of drug upon the 0–25% recovery time for the twitch response. It is found that the 0–25% recovery time is generally prolonged when the dose of vecuronium administered in the isolated forearm is increased from 0.2 to 0.6 mg; however, there is little prolongation of the 0–25% recovery interval when the dose is further increased to 2.0 mg. As a result, the delay in onset of block following administration of non-depolarizing drugs is a function of biophase binding capacity and drug affinity and, to a small extent, plasma drug concentration. As it is proposed that recovery from neuromuscular block in the isolated forearm occurs when these binding sites are substantially empty and as the rate of emptying will also depend upon the dissociation constant of the drug from these binding sites, it follows that onset and recovery are both fundamentally related to the same constant.[6] This explains the close correlation between onset time and recovery and potency which was first demonstrated by Waser,[13] Kopman[14] and Bowman et al.[16]

In order to explain the rapid onset of depolarizing block it is necessary to propose that these drugs do not become biophase-bound in the same manner as non-depolarizing agents. This is in accord with the hypothesis that we propose which suggests that a major part of depolarizing block is the result of a presynaptic action[21,22] (Chapter 14). Evidently there are no biophase binding sites to protect the presynaptic nicotinic receptors. This would also explain the difficulty of labelling these sites with a radioactive tag, and the difficulty of finding a specific ligand with a high affinity for the receptors which would allow their separation and identification. It would account for the failure of the block produced in the isolated forearm by C_{10} to increase once the tourniquet is released, why onset and recovery of depolarizing drugs do not show the same relationship as is found with non-depolarizing drugs and why recovery from depolarizing block is hastened by increasing the blood flow. It would therefore be expected that they would not show a relationship between potency and onset time.

If one accepts that the presynaptic nicotonic receptors do not have biophase binding sites, this would explain why the two non-depolarizing drugs rocuronium and ANQ9040 that demonstrate marked TOF fade during onset suggesting that they have an early presynaptic action have faster onset times than other aminosteroid drugs that demonstrate little TOF fade during onset. It would also account for the different relationship between the onset and recovery time found with rocuronium compared to other non-deploarizing drugs. This strongly suggests that the fast onset is associated with an additional, possibly presynaptic action. Further evidence to support this view is that the onset time of similar doses of rocuronium differs according to the rate or mode of stimulation by which it is measured. At 0.1 Hz the onset time of 600 μg/kg rocuronium is about 90 s.[23] If the TOF stimulation is used it is 60 s,[24] but if a 1 Hz stimulation is used then the onset time to complete block is about 45 s[6] (see Chapter 16).

In the rat phrenic nerve diaphragm preparation England et al. found that the Q_{10} for the onset of vecuronium and mivacurium neuromuscular block was between 2.4 and 2.8, suggesting that an active process involving a change in entropy underlies the onset of non-depolarizing block. This high Q_{10} is not found with C_{10}.[25] It is likely therefore that the kinetics of the onset of non-depolarizing block differs fundamentally from that of depolarizing drugs and it is the influence of the postsynaptic binding compartment that causes the slow onset of action of non-depolarizing blocking drugs.

References

1. Munday IT & Jones RM. ANQ 9040 effect of twice the ED_{95} dose. *Br J Anaesth* 1993; **70:** 480

2. Wierda JMKH, de Witt APM, Kuizenga K & Agoston S. Clinical observations on the neuromuscular blocking action of Org 9426, a steroidal non-depolarizing agent. *Br J Anaesth* 1990; **64:** 521–523

3. Waud BE. Serum *d*-tubocurarine concentration and twitch height. *Anesthesiology* 1975; **43:** 381–382

4. Lant AF. (1974) Factors affecting the action of drugs. In: *Scientific Foundations of Anaesthesia.* Scurr CF & Feldman SA (eds). London: Heinemann Medical, p. 415

5. Feldman SA, Fauvel NJ & Harrop-Griffiths W. (1970) The onset of neuromuscular blockade. In: *Neuromuscular Blocking Agents, Past, Present and Future.* Bowman WC, Denissen PAF & Feldman SA (eds). Amsterdam: Excerpta Medica, pp. 44–52

6. Feldman SA & Khaw K. The effect of variations in dose on the action of rocuronium with observations on the effect of the rate of stimulation. *Eur J Anaesthesiol* 1995; **11S:** 15–18

7. Lenter C. (ed.) (1990) *Geigy Scientific Tables* **5:** 222

8. Nigrovic V. Plasma drug concentrations: description and interpretation of the bi-experimental decay. *Br J Anaesth* 1993; **71:** 908–914

9. Goat VA, Yeung ML, Blackeney C & Feldman SA. The effect of blood flow upon the activity of gallamine triethiodide. *Br J Anaesth* 1976; **48:** 69–73

10. Feldman SA, Soni N & Kraayenbrink MA. Effect of rate of injection on the neuromuscular block produced by vecuronium. *Anesth Analg* 1989; **69:** 624–626

11. Healy TEJ, Pugh ND, Kay B *et al.* Atracurium and vecuronium: effect of dose on onset time. *Br J Anaesth* 1986; **58:** 620–624

12. Waser PG. (1966) Die Pharmakologie der Calebassenalkaloide. In: *Curare Symposium.* Waster PG (ed.). Basel: Schwabe, p. 486

13. Waser PG. Receptor localization by autoradiographic techniques. *Ann NY Acad Sci* 1967; **114:** 737–752

14. Kopman AF. Pancuronium, gallamine and *d*-tubocurarine compared: is speed of onset inversely related to potency? *Anesthesiology* 1989; **77:** 915–920

15. Lawmin JC, Bekavac I, Glavinovic MI, Donati F & Bevan DR. Iontophoretic study of speed of action of various muscle relaxants. *Anesthesiology* 1992; **77:** 351–356

16. Bowman WC, Rodger IW, Houston J *et al.* Structure: action relationship between some desacetoxy analogues of pancuronium and vecuronium in the anaesthetized cat. *Anesthesiology* 1988; **69:** 57–62

17. Kim SY, Hwang KH, Ok SY *et al.* Discrepancy of recovery times related to potency between atracurium and mivacurium simultaneously administered in isolated forearms. *Anaesthesia* 1995; **50:** 507–509

18. Feldman SA, Wu X & England AJ. Rate of onset and offset of four non-depolarizing neuromuscular blocking drugs. *Anaesthesia* 1995; **50:** 570–513

19. England AJ, Panikkar K, Redai I *et al.* Onset–offset relationship. Is rocuronium an exception? *Eur J Anaesthesiol* (in press)

20. Hood JR, Campkin NTA & Feldman SA. Curare modification of suxamethonium blockade. *Anaesthesia* 1994; **49:** 682–685

21. Feldman SA. Depolarizing neuromuscular block – a presynaptic mechanism. *Acta Anaesthesiol Scand* 1994; **38:** 535–541

22. Standaert F. They won't go away? *Acta Anaesthesiol Scand* 1994; **38:** 533–534

23. Cooper R, Mirakhur RK, Clarke RSJ & Boules Z. Comparison of intubating conditions after administering ORG 9426 (rocuronium) and suxamethonium. *Br J Anaesth* 1992; **69:** 269–273

24. Cooper R, Mirakhur RK & Maddini VR. Neuromuscular effects of rocuronium bromide (Org 9426) during fentanyl anaestheisa. *Anaesthesia* 1993; **48:** 103–105

25. England AJ, Wu X, Richards K, Redai I & Feldman SA. The influence of cold on the recovery of 3 neuromuscular blocking agents in man. *Anaesthesia* (in press)

10

Presynaptic nicotinic receptors

In 1961 Koelle[1] suggested that acetylcholine (ACh) acted both as a neuro-transmitter at postjunctional receptors and also at prejunctional sites on the motor nerve ending. In the following year Ostuka et al.[2] published a paper postulating a presynaptic mechanism to explain the depression of neuromuscular conduction by neuromuscular blocking drugs, challenging the accepted view that neuromuscular block was entirely due to their action at postsynaptic nicotinic receptors. Hubbard et al.[3] produced convincing evidence of a presynaptic effect of tubocurare in 1969 and set the scene for a detailed re-examination of occurrences that had previously been explained exclusively in terms of postsynaptic receptor activity. Over the past 30 years it has become increasingly accepted that all the neuro-muscular blocking drugs have the potential to affect presynaptic and post-synaptic receptors.[4] Thus, even α-bungarotoxin, essentially a postsynaptic receptor blocking drug, will in sufficient doses cause a decrease in ACh output and hexamethonium, considered to be essentially a presynaptic blocker, will in a dose that causes over 70% T_4/T_1 train-of-four (TOF) fade, produce a significant T_1 depression, indicating its action at the post-synaptic cholinoceptor – an observation supported by other experimental observations.[5] Much of the experimental evidence in support of the action of the non-depolarizing drugs on presynaptic nicotinic receptors comes from the simple unambiguous experiments from Bowman's group in Strathclyde[6,7] and Wessler in Germany,[8] whilst Riker,[9] Standaert and Adams[10] and Galindo[11] have produced strong evidence for a presynaptic action of the depolarizing drugs.

The evidence advanced by the Strathclyde group to support the concept of a presynaptic nicotinic receptor was that, whilst tubocurare caused neuromuscular block and tetanic fade, α-bungarotoxin produced block with minimum fade, and hexamethonium, a drug acting principally on presynaptic receptors, produced fade but little block. Wessler and his co-workers measured the output of labelled ACh and demonstrated a reduced output following a modest dose of tubocurare.[8]

The observation that tubocurare, but not vecuronium, caused an initial increase in ACh output following motor nerve activity has led to the suggestion that there are at least two populations of presynaptic receptors, each subserving different physiological functions. One group of receptors acts as a positive feedback that responds to high concentrations of ACh following motor nerve activity and the other as a negative feedback to prevent ACh mobilization in response to the background leakage of low concentrations of ACh in the absence of motor nerve activity.

Recent work in our unit has demonstrated that the onset time of the neuromuscular blocking effect of rocuronium is related to the rate of stimulation.[12] Stimulating one arm of a patient at 1 Hz gave an onset time for rocuronium that was approximately half that at 0.1 Hz. This effect is also found – albeit less marked – with vecuronium. However, the rate of stimulation does not significantly affect the recovery rate following an ED_{95} dose. We have demonstrated a similar effect in the rat phrenic nerve diaphragm preparation with vecuronium and rocuronium. However, the effect of increasing the stimulation rate is most marked after hexamethonium, which acts principally at presynaptic receptors and is not seen with α-bungarotoxin which has little, if any, presynaptic effect in the dose used.

Certainly the presence of presynaptic nicotinic receptors responding to ACh with a positive feedback mechanism increasing ACh mobilization (n_{mob}) fits the pattern of observed events and makes good teleological sense. Stimulation of such a mechanism would increase the ACh output in order to meet the demands of sustained tetanic stimulation and blockade of this system would produce tetanic fade and muscle weakness. This is especially evident when there is some postsynaptic depression produced either by drugs or disease. The increased output of ACh resulting from this positive feedback can be demonstrated to occur and its magnitude measured.[13] As a result it has become accepted that the demonstration of tetanic fade, 50 or 100 Hz for 5 s, can be taken as evidence of a block of the presynaptic receptors.[7,14] It is a short step from this assumption to propose that TOF fade is a manifestation of the same phenomenon[15] (Fig. 10.1). It has also been suggested that a separate class of presynaptic nicotinic receptors exists which promotes rapid axonal transmission and that stimulation of these receptors (n_{rep}) is responsible for the repetitive afterdischarge and antidromic firing produced by depolarizing drugs.[14]

Many workers, including myself, have no difficulty in accepting this convention as it makes possible a sensible interpretation of many clinical observations. However, it is important to appreciate that this is an assumption based on circumstantial evidence and that alternative explanations

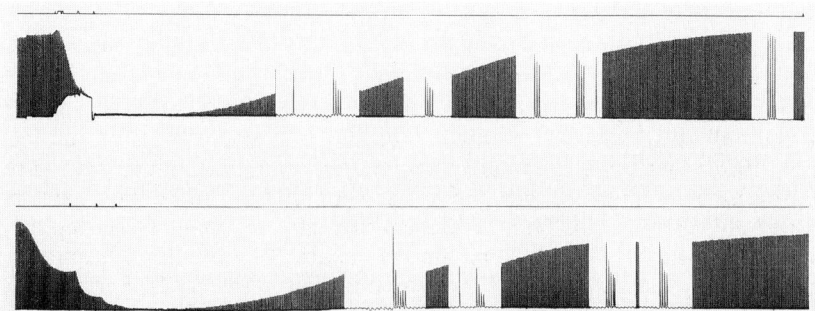

Fig. 10.1 Train-of-four fade parallels the recovery from vecuronium block in isolated arm (top trace) and after bolus injection (lower trace).

may be possible. The reason for this caution is that, in spite of all efforts, no presynaptic nicotinic receptor has been isolated. The position and composition of the structure remain unknown. This is largely due to the lack of high-affinity specific ligands but nevertheless, its presence remains unproven. It is likely to be a simpler structure than the postsynaptic cholinoceptor and may have much in common with the pentameric ganglionic nicotinic receptors. It is known that the central nervous system and autonomic ganglia lack the gene for expression of γ, δ and ε subunits and that any receptor would therefore be likely to be less complex, being composed entirely of α and β subunits, than that at the postsynaptic membrane. In general, with this class of receptor it would be anticipated that the presynaptic receptor would act as an ion gate mechanism facilitating the passage of ions. If it has characteristics similar to ganglionic nicotinic receptors then it is likely that agents such as tubocurare would more readily act as channel blockers at this site than at postsynaptic receptor sites.

It is interesting to speculate that it may be because of the simple structure of this putative receptor that drugs acting at this site lack the high-affinity binding that we postulate exists for the complex postsynaptic cholinoceptor with its greater variety of subunits. It has been demonstrated that the γ subunit alters the affinity of the neighbouring α unit 100-fold and it might be anticipated that the absence of γ and ε subunits would decrease the affinity of the presynaptic pentamer for all non-depolarizing drugs. This would also explain the difficulty of finding a specific high-affinity ligand necessary for the isolation of the receptor *in vitro*. A hypothetical but attractive phylogenetic explanation is that during evolution survival depended upon protecting the postsynaptic receptor from amines and peptides in the environment and that this resulted in a modification and specialization of the subunits of the pentamer occurring at the postjunctional receptor site in order to bind these toxins and protect muscle activity. Such a mechanism would be unnecessary to protect the prejunctional sites, which only subserve a modulating influence on ACh release. Until the presynaptic receptor is demonstrated and characterized, uncertainty as to whether or not the ACh feedback mechanism is receptor-mediated will remain.

A further caution remains in interpreting the TOF fade as evidence of presynaptic block.[16] It is difficult to understand why it occurs as quickly as at the second stimulation in the TOF. One would have anticipated the normal excess ACh production to reach only subthreshold levels after several stimulations, when a rundown of the available ACh would be significant. Indeed, Wessler[13] failed to demonstrate any decrease in ACh output following partial curarization until 10–15 stimulations were given (Fig. 10.2). Similarly, it is surprising that neostigmine, given to reverse neuromuscular block at the end of an operation, should not have an immediate action upon fade before causing any reversal of the depth of block. In practice, T_1 recovery almost invariably precedes a significant reduction in the TOF fade. It is also puzzling why the TOF fade ratio should be such a reliable guide to reversal of neuromuscular block irrespective of the drug used, when it is believed that each drug has a very different profile with respect to the presynaptic component of its action. The train

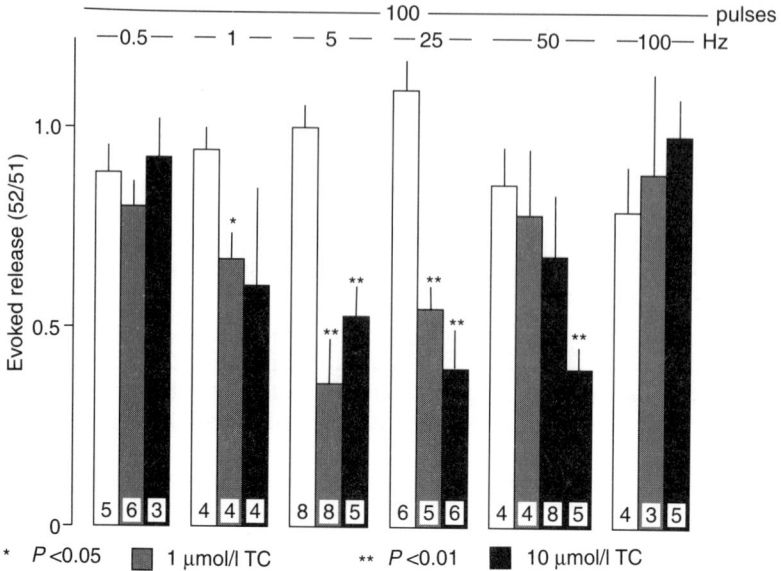

Fig. 10.2 Inhibitory effect of tubocurare (TC) on H^3 acetylcholine release following 100 pulses at 0.5–100 Hz frequency. After Wessler.[13]

of 2 Hz stimulation was initially introduced by Roberts and Wilson[18] as a test for myasthenia gravis and only introduced into anaesthesia by Ali *et al.* in 1971.[17] It remains to explain why a disease involving production of postsynaptic receptor antibodies and a diminution in postsynaptic receptor population should cause a phenomenon we have come to regard as primarily presynaptic.

Until such time as presynaptic receptors are morphologically identified and their nature and position demonstrated on the motor nerve terminal, or until stimulation by ACh is demonstrated to produce an electrical response, or an ion flux across the nerve terminal membrane, the evidence of presynaptic nicotinic receptor remains circumstantial. However, unless an alternative better explanation of observed events is advanced, it is sensible not to discard the concept for lack of definitive proof.[16]

References

1. Koelle GB. A proposed dual role of acetylcholine: its function at the pre and postsynaptic sites. *Nature* 1961; **190**: 208–211

2. Ostuka M, Endo M & Nonamura Y. Presynaptic nature of neuromuscular depression. *Jp J Physiol* 1962; **12**: 573–584

3. Hubbard JL, Wilson DF & Miyamato M. Reduction of transmitter release by *d*-tubocurarine. *Nature* 1969; **223**: 531

4. Foldes FF. (1957) In: *Muscle Relaxants in Anesthesiology*. Springfield, Ill.: Charles C Thomas

5. Redai I, Richards K, England AJ & Feldman SA. (1995) Isobolographic analysis of the interaction between hexamethonium, decamethonium and vecuronium. In: *Muscle Relaxants*, eds Fukushima and Ochiai. Tokyo: Springer-Verlag, p. 360

6. Bowman WC & Webb SN. Tetanic fade during partial transmission failure produced by non-depolarizing neuromuscular blocking drugs in the cat. *Clin Exp Pharmacol Physiol* 1976; **3:** 545–555

7. Gibb AJ & Marshall IG. Examination of the mechanism involved in tetanic fade produced by vecuronium and related analogues in rat diaphragm. *Br J Pharmacol* 1987; **90:** 511–521

8. Wessler I. Presynaptic neuromuscular block. *Anaesth Pharmacol Rev* 1993; **1:** 69–77

9. Riker WF. (1975) Prejunctional effects of neuromuscular blocking and facilitatory drugs. In: *Muscle Relaxants*. Katz RL (ed.). Monographs in Anesthesiology Series North Holland, pp. 59–102

10. Standaert FG & Adams JE. The actions of succinylcholine on motor nerve terminals. *J Pharmacol Exp Ther* 1965; **149:** 118-123

11. Galindo A. Depolarizing neuromuscular block. *J Pharmacol Exp Ther* 1971; **178:** 339–346

12. Feldman SA & Khaw K. Effect of dose of rocuronium on onset of action: observations on effect of rate of stimulation. *Eur J Anaesthesiol* 1995; **12:** 15–19

13. Wessler I. Control of transmitter release from motor nerve by presynaptic nicotinic and muscarinic receptors at the neuromuscular junction. *Trends Pharmacol Sci* 1989; **10:** 110–115

14. Bowman WC, Marshall IG, Gibb AJ *et al.* Feedback control of transmitter release at the neuromuscular junction. *Trends Pharmacol Sci* 1988; **9:** 16–20

15. Bowman WC. (1990) *Pharmacology of Neuromuscular Function*. London: Wright

16. Feldman SA. Second thoughts on the train of four. *Anaesthesia* 1993; **48:** 1–2

17. Ali HH, Utting JE & Gray CT. Quantitative assessment of residual antidepolarizing block. *Br J Anaesth* 1971; **43:** 478–485

18. Roberts RB & Wilson AT. (1968) *Myasthenia Gravis*. London: Heinemann Medical, p. 14

11

Reversing the action of non-depolarizing drugs

Anaesthetists reversing the residual effects of non-depolarizing neuro-muscular block by means of an anticholinesterase have become used to the slow improvement in twitch response and the slower recovery of the T_4/T_1 ratio following train-of-four (TOF) stimulation. Although the rate of recovery varies according to the drug used and the initial twitch height – or, more accurately, the plasma drug concentration at the time of giving the anticholinesterase, whether it be edrophonium or neostigmine – few would question the mechanism of the reversal. There is good evidence of the effectiveness of both edrophonium and neostigmine in blocking the enzymatic activity of acetylcholinesterase in the synaptic cleft and also the cholinesterase in the plasma. As a result, the normal rapid hydrolysis of acetylcholine (ACh) is reduced so that more molecules of the transmitter reach the postsynaptic membrane and, instead of the normal short half-life, the duration of life of each molecule in the proximity of the receptor is greatly enhanced. The net result is a rapid build-up of ACh from the first neural stimuli and hence a rapid decrease in the antagonist/agonist ratio and effective reversal of competitive block. This should reach its maximum effectiveness in a relatively short time, as it is the sum of the time taken for inhibition of acetylcholinesterase and the number of motor nerve discharges necessary to achieve a new higher equilibrium of ACh, which will be the result of a balance between the release of ACh and the rate of loss from the synapse as a result of diffusion into the extracellular fluid (ECF). Certainly, if intravenous edrophonium is given to treat myasthenia gravis, its maximum effect is seen within 2–3 min. It remains surprising, therefore, that it may take 5–28 min to reverse a similar weakness induced by a non-depolarizing relaxant.[1]

A second cause of surprise is why, when neostigmine is administered to reverse a residual non-depolarizing block, T_1 should be reversed at a faster rate than T_4 if TOF stimulation is used. It might have been antici-pated that the lack of ACh demonstrated by the small T_4 twitch would have been rapidly overcome by the ACh sparing produced by the anticholinesterase. If, in place of the anticholinesterase, a long-acting ACh-like agonist is administered, the T_4 fade is rapidly reversed even before T_1 reached full response. Why then does the anticholinesterase not produce the same effect as the ACh whose hydrolysis it prevents?

There is good evidence that both neostigmine and edrophonium also act as agonist drugs at the presynaptic nicotinic receptor sites – an effect independent of any ACh feedback mechanism.[2,3] A transient increase in twitch response due to both drugs can be demonstrated in the absence of twitch depression. If the dose of neostigmine is increased, in the absence of residual non-depolarizing relaxant, then ultimately neostigmine block is produced. This is particularly easily demonstrated in myasthenic patients who become increasingly resistant to anticholinesterase therapy as a result. This effect of presynaptic stimulation, followed by refractoriness, often termed desensitization, can also be produced by long-term administration of ACh or its analogues. Whilst theories have been advanced as to the cause of desensitization, it remains an obscure phenomenon. It has been attributed to ion depletion[4] from the cell, changes in the lipo-protein structure around the receptor[5] or by local changes in the muscle membrane. However, it remains unclear as to why the residual minor degree of presynaptic nicotinic receptor block present at the time of clinical reversal of non-depolarizing block should prevent its occurrence.

It would therefore appear that, whilst the anticholinesterase activity of the reversal drugs is of prime importance in reversing residual block, other additional factors have to be considered.

The speed of reversal

The speed of reversal of similar degrees of block using the same non-depolarizing relaxant is dose-dependent up to a maximum rate, beyond which increasing the dose produces little additional effect. If the speed of response is plotted against dose of anticholinesterase, an asymptote is reached, at which this occurs.[6] The actual dose varies according to initial twitch height and relaxant but seldom exceeds 0.06 mg/kg for neostigmine. This is reflected by the general advice that there is little point in giving more than 5.0 mg of neostigmine to reverse neuromuscular block.

Although it is generally held that reversal is unlikely to be successful if there is no twitch response and usually succeeds if there is 10% recovery or the first two twitches of TOF are present, these are casual associations and can misrepresent the important feature, that it is the plasma level and not the twitch response that determines the ability to produce complete safe reversal of residual block. Following the administration of an anticholinesterase, the ACh level in the synaptic cleft rises to a new level after motor nerve stimulation, which is greater than that before cholines-terase activity was blocked. This produces more effective competition with any molecules of non-depolarizing drug at the ACh receptor (AChR). It reduces the effectiveness of the antagonist drug to a level where the more ACh-sensitive fibres will contract, hence reducing the block. However, so long as drug is being released at the AChR, as a result of dis-sociation from biophase binding sites, then the reversal will be incomplete. Complete reversal depends upon substantial emptying of the biophase binding sites. This explains why it takes longer for reversal to occur than would be anticipated from a simple agonist/antagonist relationship.[7] If the biophase binding sites are constantly being refilled from drug in the plasma, then the time for emptying this reservoir increases in relation to the plasma concentration of drug. Indeed, if the plasma level is too high, it will prevent the biophase binding sites being lowered to a level that permits recovery. This explains the failure of neostigmine to cause more than a temporary reversal of the action of the non-depolarizing relaxant, when the plasma level is too high – an effect difficult to reconcile with simple competition at the AChR.[8] It explains why increasing the dose of anticholinesterase beyond maximum does not effect more effective or speedier reversal in these circumstances. It also demonstrates why it is the plasma concentration of drug rather than the twitch response that determines the ability of the anticholinesterase drugs to reverse residual neuromuscular block.

In a series of experiments to test this hypothesis, Feldman and Agoston[9] administered mixtures of neostigmine and curare in the isolated arm. Doses of 0.5 mg neostigmine together with 0.5, 1.0 or 2.0 mg of tubocurare were given in the isolated arm. The dose of neostigmine used (about 20% of a clinical reversal dose) should have produced maximum anticholinesterase effect, allowing an accumulation of ACh in the synapse and so preventing the blocking effect of the tubocurare. The experiment was designed to try and simulate *in vitro* dose ratio experiments using the isolated arm in place of the water bath of the phrenic nerve diaphragm preparation. Surprisingly, mixing neostigmine with tubocurare did not affect either the rate of onset of block or the amount of block produced. It had a marginal effect on the recovery rate of the block. This was very different from the effect of a 2.5 mg dose of neostigmine administered systemically after release of the tourniquet; in these circumstances reversal of the tubocurare block was rapid. If the systemic dose of neostigmine was administered before the isolated arm experiment was performed, virtually full block occurred rapidly in the isolated arm, although the neostigmine was administered in a dose and at a time that had previously been demonstrated to be effective in reversing the block (Fig. 11.1). These experimental results cannot be readily explained on the basis of simple competition between ACh and antagonist at the AChR.

However, if one accepts the presence of high-affinity binding sites for tubocurare near the receptor, it can be understood how the increased ACh concentration can be matched in the isolated arm by an increased drug concentration resulting from the cumulative effect of progressive dissociation of drug from binding sites. As a result, neuromuscular block ensues in spite of the increased ACh concentration. This experiment demonstrated the importance of a low plasma drug concentration at the time of reversal of non-depolarizing block by an anticholinesterase drug.

Effect of anticholinesterase on TOF

The failure of neostigmine to reverse T_4 more readily than T_1 remains difficult to explain unless one accepts a more significant presynaptic component to the action of these drugs. If the drugs were to have a clinically significant presynaptic component to their reversal action, then a residual presynaptic blocking effect of the non-depolarizing relaxant would be

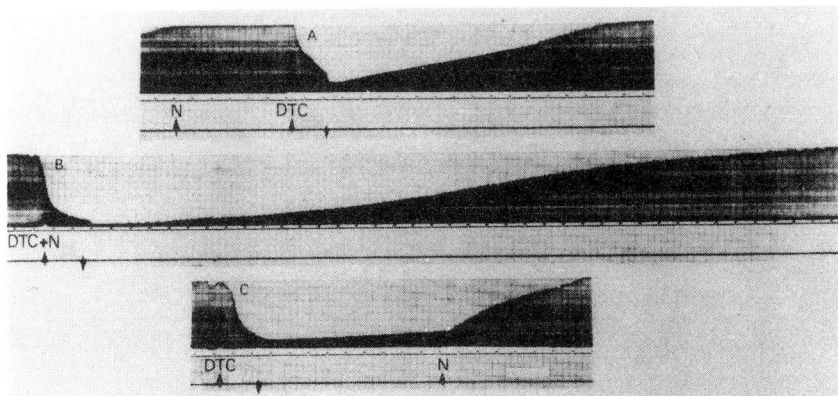

Fig. 11.1 Administration of 2 mg tubocurare (DTC) with 0.5 mg neostigmine (N) in the isolated arm did not prevent the onset of full neuromuscular block (middle trace). Neostigmine 2.5 mg administered before tubocurare in the isolated arm also did not prevent tubocurare block (upper trace). Giving the neostigmine after release of the tourniquet hastened recovery from the block (lower trace).

likely to be maintained and the effectiveness of the anticholinesterase would be diminished. The view that there is a clinically significant pre-synaptic action is supported by the ability of the residual presynaptic block of most non-depolarizing drugs to prevent neostigmine-induced presynaptic desensitization and neostigmine block.

Neostigmine or edrophonium

It has been demonstrated that edrophonium reverses residual neuro-muscular block more quickly than neostigmine in most circumstances. However, the degree of reversal is often incomplete and not infrequently followed by a minor secondary twitch depression. The more rapid onset of reversal may be related to the rather greater dose of edrophonium usually administered (in terms of ED_{50}) in order to balance its more rapid plasma clearance.[10] However, it is possible that it is caused by the different method of producing its anticholinesterase effect (see Chapter 4). It is a common observation that edrophonium is less effective at causing a per-manent reversal of major degrees of block. Typically, if a large dose of edrophonium is given at less than 10% recovery of twitch response the reversal, although rapid, will start to fail after 2–3 min, leaving some residual block. It is tempting to suggest that this early effective reversal is due to a transitory presynaptic effect causing a release of ACh; as this wanes, the ratio of ACh to drug in the synaptic cleft is reduced and some block recurs.

Other factors that have been demonstrated to reduce the rate of block reversal by anticholinesterase drugs include low cardiac output, low blood flow and the presence of greater than minimum alveolar concentrations of anaesthetic vapours.[11,12] Reduced renal blood flow, hepatic disease and jaundice – especially if aminosteroid relaxants have been used – may also

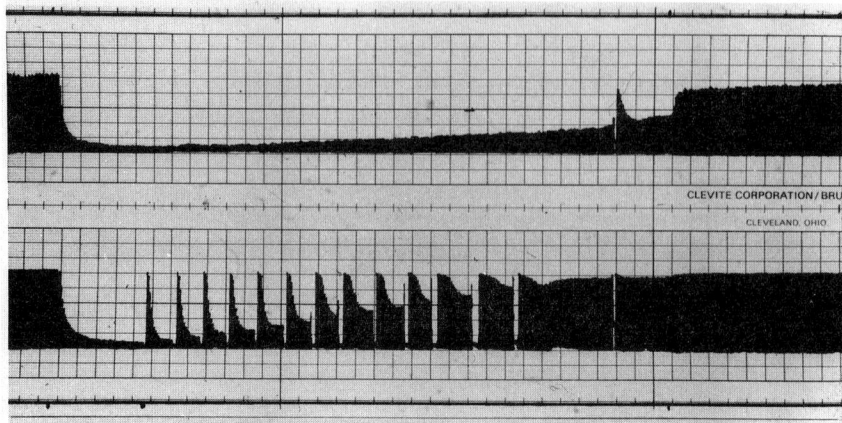

Fig. 11.2 Repeat tetanic contractions of the hand increase the rate of reversal of tubocurare neuromuscular block in patients (lower trace). Central hand (upper trace).

delay reversal by prolonging the normal metabolism and excretion of the drugs and so prevent the low plasma concentration of antagonist essential for reversal by an anticholinesterase. A low plasma cholinesterase level will markedly prolong the action of mivacurium and prevent its reversal by anticholinesterase.

Although many causes of failure of neostigmine to reverse the action of antagonist block have been suggested,[13–15] in practice nearly all such occurrences are examples of a failure to reduce the plasma level of drug sufficiently at the time of reversal. Indeed, in the presence of low plasma concentrations of drug, ACh released by repeated tetanic stimulation is itself sufficient to produce early reversal (Fig. 11.2). This explains the more rapid recovery of diaphragmatic movement in patients with normal or raised carbon dioxide levels compared to patients who are hyperventilated. In the former groups, high-frequency phrenic nerve activity will produce early reversal of the block at the diaphragm.

The syndrome of neostigmine-resistant curarization described by Hunter[13] has been attributed not solely to the inability of neostigmine to reverse the neuromuscular block but also to a concomitant serious base deficit producing a metabolic acidosis due to the patient's inability to hyperventilate in order to compensate for the low buffer base.[16] It is the acidaemia that causes the unconsciousness, tracheal tug and a failure of the low blood pressure to respond to catecholamines and not the residual curarization.[17]

References

1. Savarese JJ. Reversal of non-depolarizing blocks: more controversial than ever? *Anesth Analg* 1993; Reports IARS (suppl) 78–82
2. Braga MFM, Rown EG, Harvey AL & Bowman WC. Prejunctional action of neostigmine on mouse neuromuscular preparations. *Br J Anaesth* 1993; **70:** 405–410

3. Blaber LC. The mechanism of the facilitatory action of edrophonium in the cat skeletal muscle. *Br J Pharmacol* 1972; **46:** 498

4. Madicke A. (1990) The nicotinic receptor. In: *Muscle Relaxant.* Agoston A & Bowman WC (eds). Holland: Elsevier Science, pp. 19–44

5. Prinz H. (1986) A general treatment of ligand binding to acetylcholine receptor. In: *Structure and Function of Nicotinic Acetylcholine Receptor.* Malicke A (ed.) ASI Series (H). Cell Biology, vol. 3. Berlin: Springer Verlag, pp. 129–146

6. Morris RB, Cronnely R, Miller RD *et al.* Pharmacokinetics of edrophonium and neostigmine when antagonising *d*-tubocurarine blockade in man. *Anesthesiology* 1981; **54:** 399–402

7. Feldman SA. (1979) *Muscle Relaxants.* London: WB Saunders, p. 50

8. Feldman SA & Levi AJ. Prolonged paresis following gallamine. *Br J Anaesth* 1963; **35:** 804–807

9. Feldman SA & Agoston S. Failure of neostigmine to prevent tubocurarine neuromuscular block in the isolated arm. *Br J Anaesth* 1980; **52:** 1199–1205

10. Kopman AF. The pharmacokinetics of anticholinesterase. *Anaesth Pharm Rev* 1993; **1:** 88–92

11. Bevan DR, Donati F & Kopman AF. Reversal of neuromuscular blockade. *Anesthesiology* 1992; **77:** 785–790

12. Gill SS, Bevan DR & Donati F. Edrophonium antagonism of atracurium during enflurane anaesthesia. *Br J Anaesth* 1990; **64:** 300–305

13. Hunter AR. Neostigmine resistant curarisation. *Br Med J* 1956; **11:** 919–921

14. Burchill GB. Irreversible curarisation. *Br J Anaesth* 1957; **29:** 127–128

15. Paton WDM. Possible causes of prolonged apnoea. *Anaesthesia* 1958; **13:** 253

16. Brooks DK & Feldman SA. Metabolic acidosis; a new approach to neostigmine resistant curarisation. *Anaesthesia* 1962; **17:** 161–165

17. Feldman SA. (1974) The significance of acid base balance. In: *Scientific Foundations of Anaesthesia.* Scurr CF & Feldman SA (eds). London: Heinemann Medical, pp. 397–402

12

Sensitivity to a second drug dose

The margin of safety theory and the iceberg

In 1967 Paton and Waud[1] produced a paper on the margin of safety of neuromuscular transmission that had a profound effect upon our interpretation of the events occurring during clinical neuromuscular block. The starting point of their investigation was to relate the degree of twitch depression in a muscle to the amount of receptor blockade. They estimated the effect of competition at the receptor in terms of receptor occlusion. This was calculated from the ratio of agonist to antagonist drug necessary to reduce end-plate depolarization by a set amount after motor nerve stimulation. In their experiments they used various agonists (including suxamethonium) and antagonists (tubocurare and gallamine). They reasoned that the choice of agonist and antagonist should not matter, on the assumption that these drugs only act postsynaptically, that tubocurare and suxamethonium both compete for the same receptor on the post-synaptic membrane and that block of this receptor alone by tubocurare will produce failure of neuromuscular transmission. We now know that both suxamethonium and tubocurare have significant presynaptic actions[2,3] and that suxamethonium may have a long-acting depressing effect on acetylcholine (ACh) release presynaptically after a brief stimulation.[4] The assumption that both tubocurare and suxamethonium compete for the same receptor site is solidly based on the law of mass action but it ignores the possibility that in addition tubocurare may bind to other non-active acceptor sites[5] – biophase binding – and that the bound drug would not be free to compete with agonist.

Paton and Waud found from calculations based on the results of their log dose response studies, that a fractional receptor occupancy of 76% was required before any block of indirectly elicited muscle response could be demonstrated and 91% occupancy before full block occurred (Fig. 12.1). They also observed that the interaction of the agonist and antagonist when tested over a wide range of dosages did not fully conform to conditions for competitive equilibrium. At higher doses the linearity of the plot was markedly distorted. They concluded that this was the result of quasiequilibrium between agonist and antagonist.

In further experiments carried out in Boston, Waud and Waud[6] elaborated upon these findings. Using a phrenic nerve diaphragm preparation,

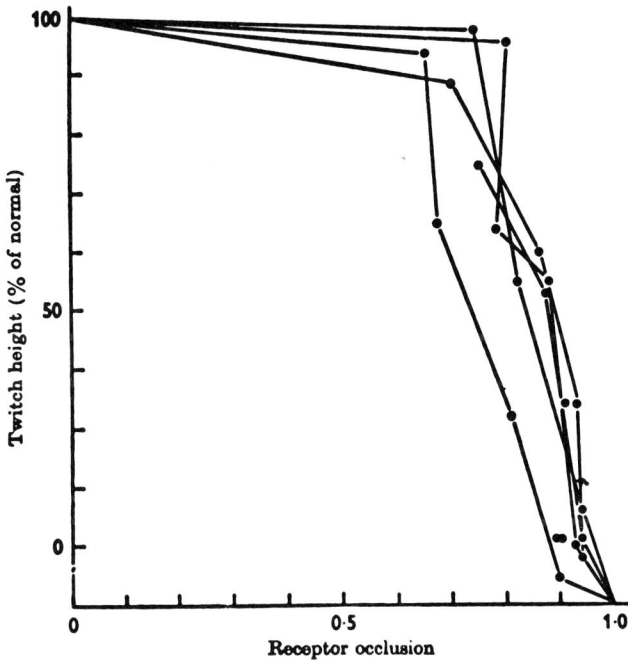

Fig. 12.1 The margin of safety of neuromuscular transmission. There is little depression of twitch response until >74% receptors are 'occupied' by drug. From Paton and Waud.[1]

they demonstrated that the margin of safety was less if tetanic stimulation was used and at 50 Hz tetanic stimulation of 100 Hz occurred at approximately 50% receptor occupancy (Fig. 12.3).

The concept of a margin of safety envisages a large pool of ACh receptors (AChR) and an excess production of ACh in response to motor nerve stimulation. ACh is thus available to activate many more receptors than is required to bring about depolarization of the end-plate; this constitutes the margin of safety. Initial estimates suggested that 300 000–500 000 ACh molecules were liberated from a single motor nerve; this is vastly in excess of the number calculated to be required to produce the end-plate current necessary for depolarization.

The margin of safety theory suggested that only when >75% of the AChR were effectively occupied* was there a restriction of AChR activation such that the end-plate current generated would be insufficient to produce threshold depolarization for the most sensitive muscle fibres, and as the antagonist drug concentration is increased, more and more muscle fibres would be blocked.

---

* The term occupation is somewhat misleading: in a dynamic process it reflects a higher random chance of reaction occurring between receptor and antagonist drug than receptor and agonist rather than physical occupancy of the receptor.

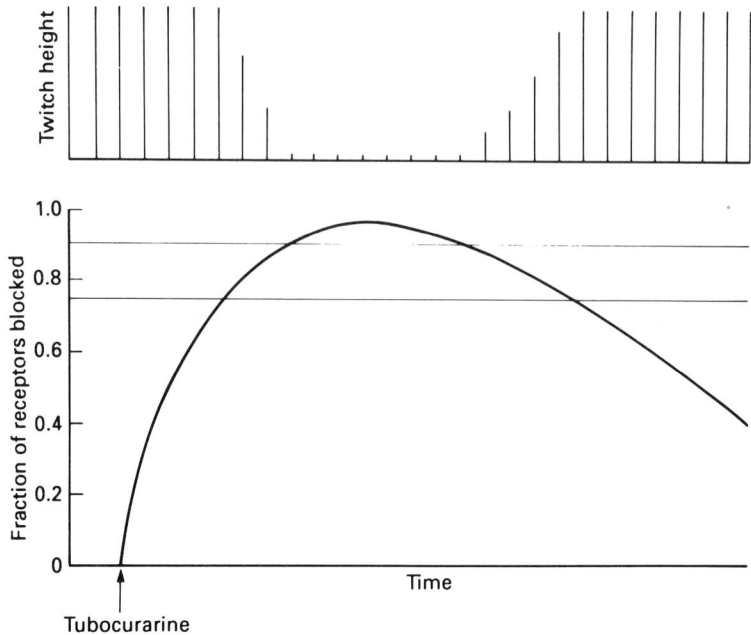

Fig. 12.2 The iceberg theory. Monitoring twitch response will only reveal >75% to <91% receptor occlusion. From Waud and Waud.[7]

This led Waud and Waud[7] to postulate the iceberg theory (Fig. 12.2). The iceberg theory suggests that, since twitch depression requires >75% receptor occupancy and full block occurs at >95% occupancy, it is impossible to measure less than 75% of residual receptor occupancy using the twitch response. This undetectable range of receptor occupation was likened to the bulk of an iceberg that lies concealed beneath the water. If, however, one uses tetanic stimulation at 50 or 100 Hz, then more of the iceberg is revealed. Even at 100 Hz stimulation, receptor occupancy of less than 50% would still remain impossible to detect.[8]

It is implicit in the margin of safety concept that at the point of complete twitch recovery there remains a considerable reservoir of occupied receptors. This concept has led to the assumption that the cause of second dose sensitivity to non-depolarizing drugs is the residual receptor occupancy and that recurarization is always possible in spite of complete recovery of the twitch response.[9] It is a similar reasoning that has been used to explain the priming effect of giving a dose of drug in two separate boluses, i.e. a small priming dose, followed at 4 min by the remainder[10,11] to produce a more rapid onset of block.

Although the overall observations of Paton and Waud[1] and Waud and Waud[7] are not seriously questioned, there is cause to doubt the interpretation that they and others have placed on these findings. It is now believed that the previous calculations of the amount of ACh released presynaptically as a result of motor nerve activity resulted in a considerable overestimate. If the number of ACh molecules released were fewer than

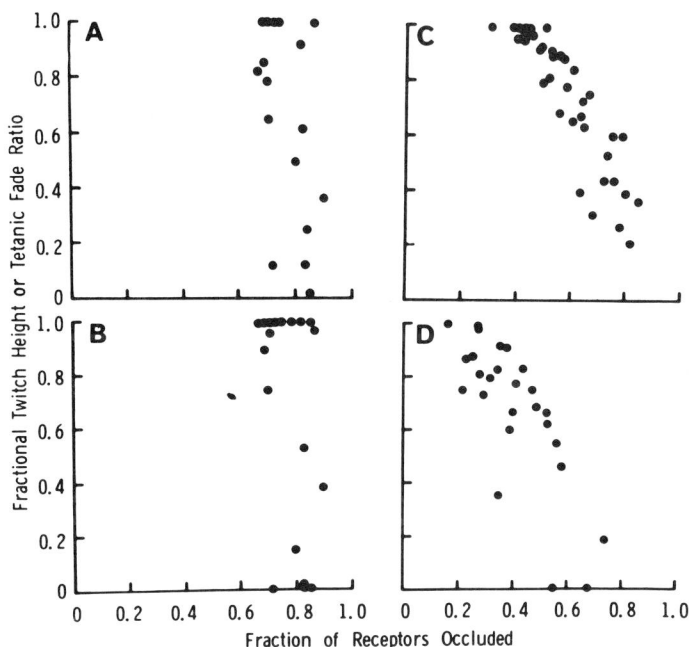

Fig. 12.3 Effect of increasing the rate of stimulation upon receptor occupancy required to produce block. A 0.1 Hz; B 30 Hz; C 100 Hz; D 200 Hz.

50 000, then there would be too few to activate a vast pool of postsynaptic AChR and neuromuscular conduction would be vulnerable at much lower concentrations of antagonist as it required only a small percentage of the receptors to be blocked by the antagonist. The acceptance of a margin of safety necessarily assumes a large excess release of ACh following motor nerve stimulation. This is now considered to be improbable in humans.

Recent evidence suggests that at recovery of twitch response there is little residual receptor occupancy. This comes from studies in the isolated forearm. Following 95% block by vecuronium, pancuronium or tubocurare it has been demonstrated that the 50 and 100 Hz tetanic fade which is present as the block diminishes cannot be demonstrated at the time of complete twitch recovery[12] (Fig. 12.4). This finding cannot be reconciled with the assumption in the iceberg theory that at the time of twitch recovery there is >75% receptor occupancy. According to Waud and Waud,[7] tetanic fade at 100 Hz should occur if there is 50% receptor occupancy. Further evidence against the iceberg theory is that at the time of twitch recovery in the isolated arm the log dose–response to vecuronium is the same as it is in the control arm and in patients who have not received any vecuronium[13] (Fig. 12.5). If there had been residual receptor occupancy one would have anticipated a considerable shift to the left of the log dose–response in the arm that had been blocked.

What then is the explanation of the apparent spare receptors for tubo-curare that Paton and Waud interpreted as the margin of safety? Our experiments suggest that, following administration of a non-depolarizing

Vecuronium
0.3mg

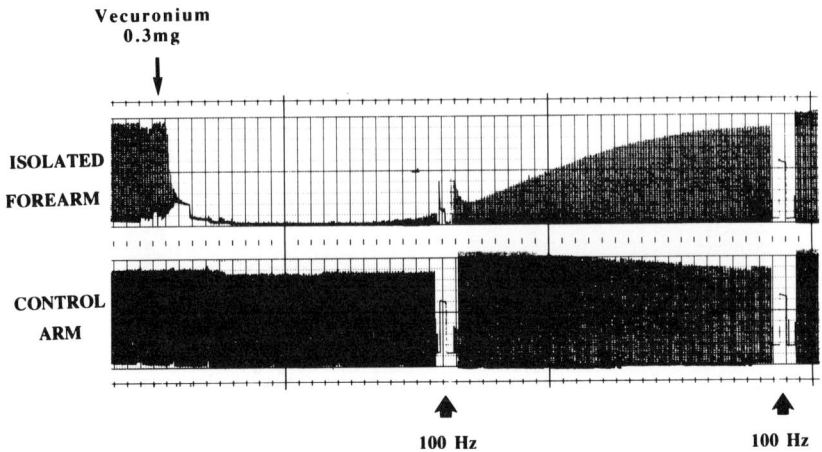

ISOLATED

FOREARM

CONTROL

ARM

100 Hz   100 Hz

Fig. 12.4 Although tetanic fade can be demonstrated at 50% recovery of the twitch response in the isolated arm, no fade can be demonstrated on recovery of neuromuscular transmission. This is inconsistent with the iceberg theory.

neuromuscular blocking drug, molecules of the drug are taken up by high-affinity binding sites in the biophase.[14] The onset of competitive action at the AChR occurs when the drug dissociates from these sites. Thus the drug with lowest affinity will have the most rapid onset (see Chapter 9). Since these binding sites will temporarily sequestrate drug molecules, they will not be available for competition with an agonist and in dose ratio experiments will appear to be extra AChRs occupied by antagonist. As such, they will not be available to compete with ACh and will not prevent ACh generating an end-plate current. They will appear to be 'spare receptors' (Fig. 12.6).

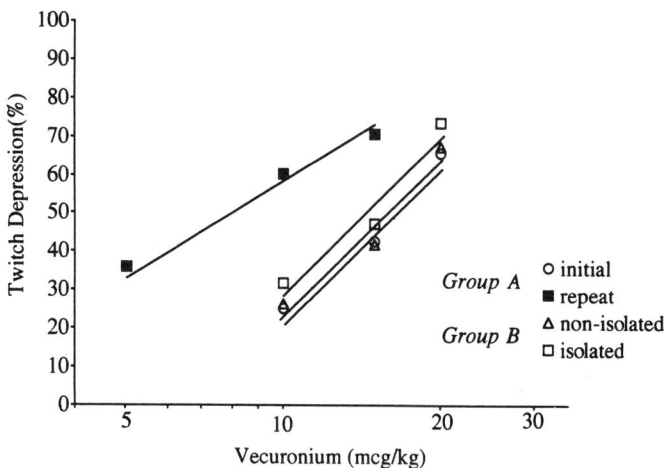

Fig. 12.5 Following recovery of the twitch response in the isolated arm, the sensitivity to a second dose of vecuronium is not statistically different from the control arm. From Campkin et al.,[13] with permission.

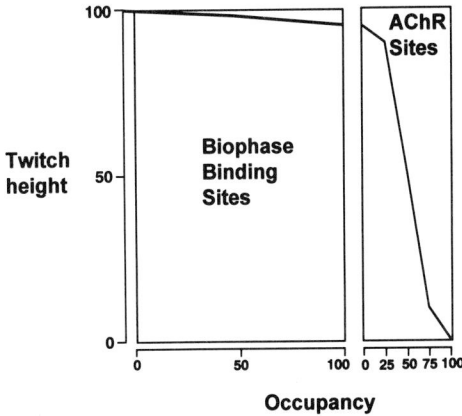

Fig. 12.6 Schematic reinterpretation of the margin of safety incorporating a biophase binding compartment. AChR = Acetylcholine receptor. It is proposed that the sequestration of drug in these binding sites gives the impression of 'spare receptors'.

If this interpretation is true, then only part of the tubocurare antagonist drug administered during the titration of agonist against antagonist in Paton and Waud's dose ratio experiments is truly competitive. This may explain their finding that there is a loss of linearity in the relationship, which the original observers suggested might be due to a state of quasi-equilibrium.

The observations of Waser[15] support the suggestion that some of the molecules of non-depolarizing drug administered initially take no part in competition with ACh at the receptor. He demonstrated that paralysis only started to develop after 50% of an ED_{95} dose of radiolabelled toxiferine had been administered and had become fixed at the postsynaptic membrane (Fig. 12.7).

Whether this theory provides a more acceptable explanation of the margin of safety findings requires further experiments. However, it is evident that the original interpretation must be seriously questioned.

The cause of second dose sensitivity

If residual receptor occupancy is not the cause of the second dose sensitivity seen when 'top-up' doses of non-depolarizing relaxants are administered, what is the cause?

Experiments carried out using mivacurium provide some clues to this puzzle. Although mivacurium is rapidly cleared from the plasma at the time of recovery of full twitch response following an ED_{95} dose, some 18–20 min after administration of the drug, the log dose–response of a second 'top-up' dose of drug is shifted to the left, revealing a 50% reduction in dose requirement. This reduction in second dose requirement is similar to that seen after vecuronium.[16] As little mivacurium will be remaining in the plasma and extracellular fluid at this time, the effect is

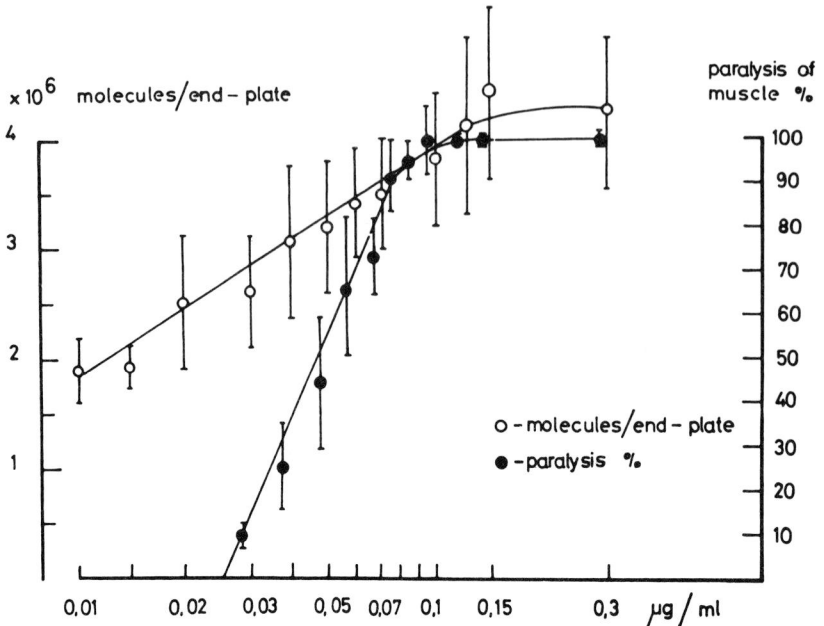

Fig. 12.7 The relationship between the molecular saturation of toxiferine and paralysis. No paralysis was observed before 50% of blocking dose was administered. From Waser,[15] with permission.

much less likely to be due to residual mivacurium at AChR or in the plasma than is the case with vecuronium.

If one arm of a patient is excluded by a tourniquet from the circulation for 3 min after the administration of an ED$_{95}$ dose of mivacurium, then upon release of the tourniquet little or no block occurs in the excluded arm. This is the basis of the bioassay method of following the fall in the effective level of drug in the blood.[17] Following recovery from the mivacurium block in the arm not excluded from the circulation by the tourniquet, a log dose–response to a second 'top-up' dose of drug reveals that both the blocked arm and the non-blocked arm demonstrate the same second dose sensitivity (Figs 12.8 and 12.9).

Clearly, the effect is not due to the presence of residual drug at the receptor or in the plasma but to a reduced distribution volume for the drug in the patient. This is hardly surprising with drugs such as tubocurare and the aminosteroids in view of autoradiographic evidence that these neuromuscular blocking drugs redistribute rapidly in high concentrations to the liver, kidney and spleen (Fig. 12.10). It remains to be seen whether this also occurs with mivacurium, whose initial distribution volume is so large that it is usually accepted that it represents the rapid hydrolysis of the drug in the plasma rather than its sequestration in the body.

It is known that once these distribution sites are filled they empty slowly. During this time they will reduce the volume of distribution of a subsequent 'top-up' dose of drug. It is evident that second dose sensitivity to top-up doses of non-depolarizing drugs does not depend upon there being

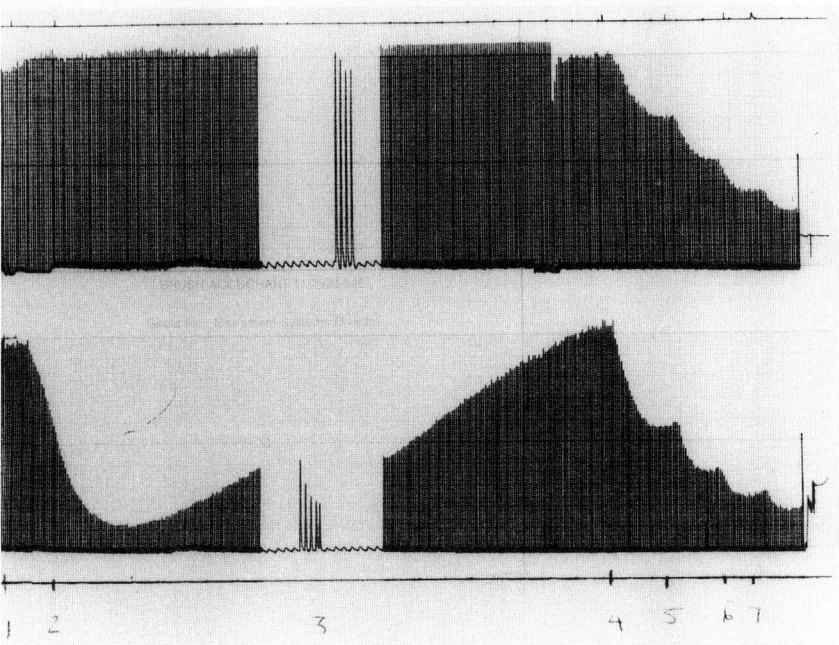

Fig. 12.8 Both the patient arm protected from ED_{95} dose of mivacurium for 3 min (upper trace) and the arm 90% blocked (lower trace) demonstrate similar sensitivity to a second mivacurium dose–response at 100% recovery of the blocked arm.

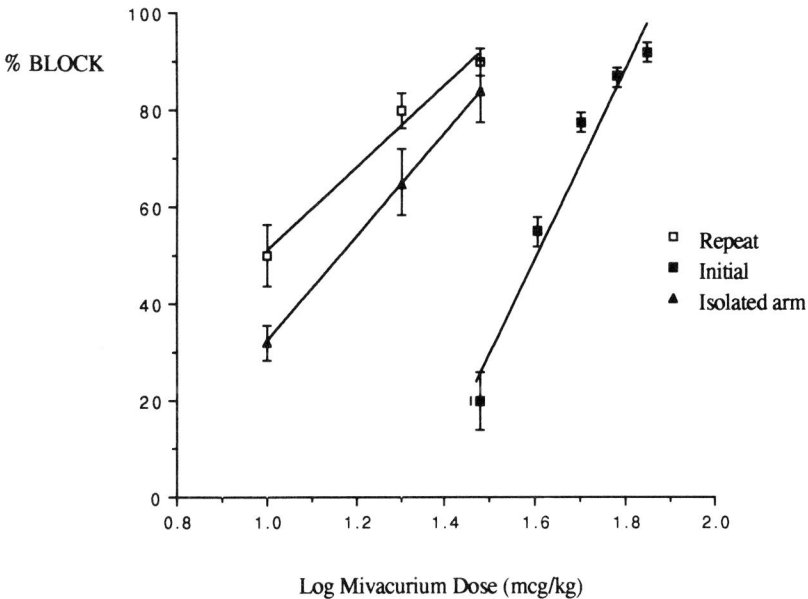

Log Mivacurium Dose (mcg/kg)

Fig. 12.9 A second dose sensitivity to mivacurium is similar in the arm excluded from the blocking concentration of drug and the arm which is 95% blocked. In both there is an approximately 50% reduction in the ED_{50}.

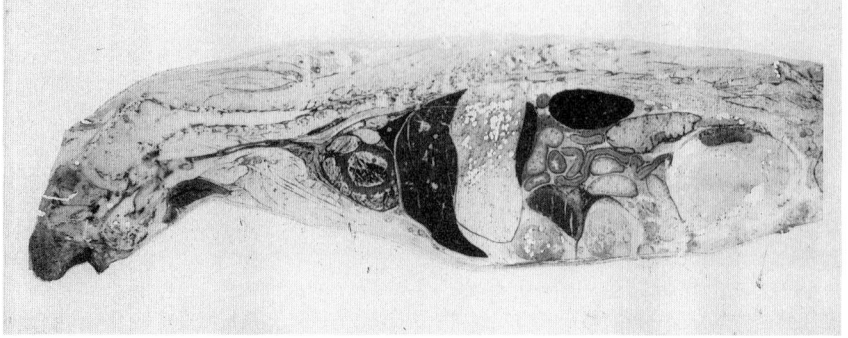

Fig. 12.10 Autoradiograph of rat 3 min after recovery from H^3 tubocurare. Note the concentration of drug in the liver and kidneys; this represents a large part of the rapid distribution volume. From Cohen et al.,[19] with permission.

an iceberg of concealed receptor occupancy. Indeed, there is strong evidence that the iceberg does not exist. There is little doubt that there is sequestration of a portion of the tubocurare dose at the synapse before agonist–antagonist competition occurs, but present evidence suggests that this is not at receptor sites but rather at biophase binding or acceptor sites, which are emptied when twitch recovery occurs.[18]

References

1. Paton WDM & Waud DR. The margin of safety of neuromuscular transmission. *J Physiol* 1967; **191:** 59–90

2. Feldman SA & Hood JR. Depolarizing neuromuscular block. A presynaptic mechanism? *Acta Anaesthesiol Scand* 1994; **38:** 535–541

3. Bowman WC. Prejunctional and postjunctional cholinoceptors at the neuromuscular junction. *Anesth Analg* 1980; **59:** 935–943

4. Galindo A. Depolarizing neuromuscular block. *J Pharmacol Exp Ther* 1971; **339:** 346

5. Feldman SA. Biophase binding: its effect on recovery from non-depolarizing neuromuscular block. *Anesth Pharm Rev* 1993; **1:** 81–88

6. Waud DR & Waud BE. The relation between tetanic fade and receptor occlusion in the presence of competitive neuromuscular block. *Anesthesiology* 1971; **35:** 456–461

7. Waud BE & Waud DR. (1975) Physiology and pharmacology of neuromuscular blocking agents. In: *Muscle Relaxants*. Katz RL (ed.). Holland: Excerpta Medica/Elsevier, pp. 1–51

8. Feldman SA. (1974) Measurements of neuromuscular block. In: *Measurements in Anaesthesia*. Spierdijk J, Feldman SA & Leigh J (eds). Holland: Leiden University Press

9. Bowman WC. (1990) In: *Pharmacology of Neuromuscular Function*. London: W Wright, pp. 170–171

10. Foldes FF, Nagashima H & Karnak PH. Effect of priming. *Anaesth Pharmacol Rev* 1993; **1:** 48–56

11. Taboada JA, Rupp SM & Miller RD. Refining the priming principle for vecuronium during rapid sequence induction of anaesthesia. *Anesthesiology* 1986; **64:** 243–247

12. Campkin NTA, Hood JR & Feldman SA. Train of four and 50 Hz tetanus during recovery from neuromuscular block. *Anesth Analg* 1993; **76:** 33

13. Campkin NTA, Hood JR, Fauvel NJ & Feldman SA. The effect of residual receptor occupancy on sensitivity to repeated vecuronium. *Anaesthesia* 1994; **48:** 572–575

14. Feldman SA. Biophase binding: its effect on recovery from non-depolarising neuro-muscular block. *Anaesth Pharmacol Rev* 1993; **1:** 81–87
15. Waser PG. (1970) On receptors in the postsynaptic membrane of the motor end plate. In: *Ciba Foundation Symposium on the Molecular Properties of Drug Receptors.* Porter R & O'Connor M (eds). London: Churchill, pp. 59–71
16. Feldman SA, Hood JR, Campkin NTA & Rehm S. Sensitivity to second dose of mivacurium. *Anaesthesia* 1994; **49:** 671–674
17. Hood JR. A mivacurium bioassay. Presented at Anaesthetic Research Society Meeting (1993), London
18. Feldman SA. (1995) The iceberg theory – fact or fiction? Implications for monitoring. In: *Muscle Relaxants*, Fukushima K & Ochiai R (eds). Tokyo: Springer-Verlag, pp. 257–262
19. Cohen EN, Hood N & Golling R. Use of whole body autoradiography for determination of uptake and distribution of labelled muscle relaxants in the rat. *Anesthesiol* 1968; **28:** 309–313

13

The priming principle

Although the administration of a small initial dose of muscle relaxant 3–4 min before the main dose was common practice by the Liverpool School of Anaesthetists in the late 1950s and early 1960s, the purpose was not to speed up the onset of block but rather to detect patients with latent myasthenia gravis. However, it is interesting to reflect that Professor Gray, the principal advocate of this technique, always claimed that the onset of intubating conditions with tubocurare, the relaxant in use at that time, was rapid.

In 1984 Foldes[1] pointed out the effect of a small initial dose of non-depolarizing drug upon the rate of onset and duration of action of a subsequent bolus dose. He termed this the priming principle and in this way the technique became established. Various studies have demonstrated particular features of this effect,[2,3] as well as focusing attention on the possible dangers associated with its use in the very patients in whom its use was most needed – those requiring early intubation to protect the trachea from aspiration of stomach contents.[4,5]

Foldes based his recommended dose regime on the observation that it was possible to give a small dose of tubocurare which caused weakness of the hand without producing any reduction in ventilatory capacity or vital capacity.[5] With these small doses the maximum effect on grip strength occurs in 4–5 min. It was reasoned that this dose represented the number of molecules required to produce marginal twitch depression. By interpolating this on the concept of margin of safety of neuromuscular transmission and the receptor occupation–twitch depression relationship,[6] it was suggested that this small dose of tubocurare, about 0.1 mg/kg, represented the dose necessary to produce about a 90% receptor occupancy. If a slightly smaller dose were used it would have little, if any, motor effect but should facilitate subsequent paralysis when a second dose of drug was administered. The technique was then developed using a fraction of the intubating dose to prime the margin of safety receptor pool, followed by the remainder of the bolus at the time when maximum effect would be anticipated, i.e. in 3–4 min. The usual intubating bolus dose of non-depolarizing blocking drug is $2–3 \times ED_{95}$ and an initial priming dose of 10% of this bolus, i.e. $0.2–0.3 \times ED_{95}$. This is the usual dose regime that has been recommended to prime patients.[3,7,8]

A contribution of a presynaptic block of nicotinic receptors to the priming effect has been suggested by Schwarz et al.[2] They observed that the more rapid onset of block by vecuronium in primed patients was accompanied by a more marked train-of-four (TOF) fade. It is interesting that although TOF fade develops after T_1 depression with large bolus doses of vecuronium and other drugs, all techniques and drugs associated with a faster onset of non-depolarizing block, no matter how it is produced, are usually associated with an increased TOF fade. It is possible that early depression of acetylcholine (ACh) release by a presynaptic blocking action reduces the margin of safety of neuromuscular transmission, so rendering early onset of block possible. However, pretreatment with Mg^{2+} to reduce ACh release has not been demonstrated to affect the speed of onset of a bolus dose of drug or to affect priming.[9]

The effectiveness of priming has been established with most non-depolarizing relaxants. However, the priming capacity of atracurium is controversial.[10–12] The recommended priming doses of vecuronium are between 5 mg and 20 μg/kg and a dose of 60 mg to 120 μg/kg[2] for tubocurare.[13] There is no advantage in exceeding these maximum values; although lower priming doses produce less effect on onset times,[14] higher priming doses do not seem to speed up the onset time. These doses nearly always produce some diplopia and in susceptible patients may produce difficulty in controlling the tongue and in swallowing. Indeed, it has been suggested that for priming to reduce the onset time to about 60 s, a priming dose that just produces difficulty in swallowing and diplopia is required.[15,16] For this reason it is generally advised that some form of sedation should be administered and the technique should not be used when there is a significant risk of the aspiration of stomach content or vomit, unless alternative techniques, such as the use of suxamethonium, carry a greater risk to the patient.[5,17]

Based on the initial observation that the time to maximum effect of the small dose of tubocurare used in the original study was 4 min, this time interval has generally been recommended and it has been confirmed that when vecuronium is used, 4 min was more effective than 2 and 6 min as a priming interval.

Not every study has confirmed the efficacy of priming for all relaxants.[11,12] Attempts to use rocuronium in this way have been largely unsuccessful in reducing the relatively rapid onset time of this drug still further. Atracurium is less effective than most non-depolarizing drugs as a priming agent and a recent study using mivacurium failed to demonstrate an effect on the relatively slow onset of this drug unless 7 min had elapsed between the two doses of drug.[18]

Recently the way in which priming causes a reduction in onset time has been studied and the assumption that it is the result of partial ACh receptor occupancy has been questioned for the following reasons:

1 It is difficult to envisage a pharmacokinetic reason to explain why giving a drug in divided doses (as happens with priming) makes it more effective than giving the whole dose rapidly as a bolus.[19] In order to accept marginal receptor occupancy by the priming dose, one would have to

assume that it takes 4 min to equilibrate the plasma, extracellular fluid (ECF) synaptic cleft and ACh receptor (AChR) drug concentration. However, at 4 min after injection of a priming dose, the plasma concentration of drug will be very low, having been partially cleared by redistribution, especially to the kidney and liver. It can only be explained if the drug became bound at the receptor site and the receptor occupancy continued minutes after the plasma ECF and synaptic cleft concentrations had fallen to levels at which very little occupation would be anticipated. However, this cannot occur if the drug–receptor retention is protean. To explain this phenomenon it is therefore necessary to invoke a biophase binding site; this is recognized in the only adequate pharmacokinetic model.[20] If such a binding site did not exist in the biophase, then priming would not occur and the remainder of the bolus dose would take longer than normal to produce neuromuscular block.

2 If the primary dose of vecuronium is administered by continuous slow infusion over the 4 min before the intubating dose, it is just as effective in reducing onset time as if the priming dose had been given as a bolus (N Hirsch, personal communication). However, when vecuronium is administered in this way the plasma concentration of vecuronium is never high enough to cause significant receptor occupancy unless a mechanism exists to concentrate or sequest the drug against its concentration gradient.

3 If the priming dose of vecuronium is given 10 min before the intubating dose, it is still almost as effective as when it is given at 4 min, yet the rapid AChR–drug reaction would be ineffective to maintain drug in the biophase for this length of time against its plasma receptor concentration gradient (Feldman, unpublished observations).

4 If a priming dose of mivacurium is given at 3 or 4 min before the intubating dose, its effect on onset time is marginal. However, when it is administered 7–10 min before the intubating dose, the onset is reduced to 60–80 s.[18] This is difficult to reconcile with the rapid clearance of this drug from the plasma.

These observations suggest that the effect of priming upon the onset of non-depolarizing block continues long after the plasma concentration of drug has fallen. In the case of the infusion experiment the efficacy of priming is demonstrated not to depend upon achieving a plasma level that produces symptoms of marginal block in sensitive tissues demonstrating 80–90% ACh receptor occupancy, but upon the total dose used in the prime. It appears that the number of drug molecules used to prime the patient is more important than the plasma concentration–synaptic cleft gradient achieved and that a mechanism exists to bind these molecules in the synapse and to maintain them close to the AChR even when the plasma concentration of drug declines. This view is compatible with the concept of a biophase binding reservoir that has a high affinity for the drug molecules. Thus, once the binding reservoir is partially filled by the drug molecules, further administration of the drug as the definitive bolus or a bolus of another non-depolarizing agent will more readily affect the AChR.

It remains to explain why rocuronium is ineffective as a priming agent before bolus doses of rocuronium. One can speculate that rocuronium in low doses acts primarily at presynaptic nicotinic receptors and that binding does not occur at this site in the same way as at postsynaptic receptors.

In a four-way cross-over study of priming we studied the effectiveness of rocuronium to prime rocuronium or vecuronium and of vecuronium to prime rocuronium.[21] It was found that rocuronium was ineffective at priming rocuronium but that vecuronium priming reduced rocuronium onset time by 50% (Fig. 13.1). Rocuronium and vecuronium both reduce the onset time of vecuronium. It is evident that rocuronium can be used as a priming agent but whatever causes its effect, it is ineffective when followed by more rocuronium as the bolus dose. This is consistent with the hypothesis that rocuronium has an early presynaptic effect and this causes its rapid onset. This additional effect would prime vecuronium but would not be useful in reducing the onset time of rocuronium itself.

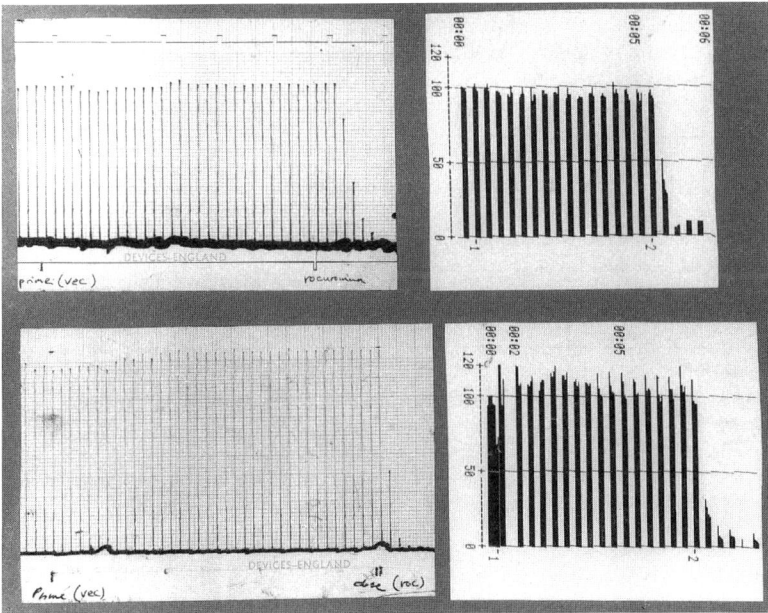

Fig. 13.1 Effectiveness of vecuronium as a priming agent for rocuronium. Left-hand panels: 0.2 Hz twitch; right-hand panels: train-of-four relaxograph trace from the opposite hand. In both experiments the onset of rocuronium block was reduced to approximately 40 s.

References

1. Foldes FF. Rapid tracheal intubation with non-depolarizing neuromuscular blocking drugs: the priming principle (letter). *Br J Anaesth* 1984; **56**: 663
2. Schwarz S, Ilias W, Lacknar R, Mayerhofer S & Foldes FF. Rapid tracheal intubation with vecuronium. The priming principle. *Anesthesiology* 1985; **62**: 388–391

3. Sosis M, Stiener A, Larijan GE & Marr AT. An evaluation of priming with vecuronium. *Br J Anaesth* 1987; **59:** 1236–1239

4. Musich J & Watts LF. Pulmonary aspiration after a priming dose of vecuronium. *Anesthesiology* 1986; **64:** 517–519

5. Donati F. The priming saga – where do we stand now? *Can J Anaesth* 1988; **35:** 1–4

6. Foldes FF, Nagashima H & Karnak PM. Effect of priming. *Anaesth Pharmacol Rev* 1993; **1:** 49–56

7. Mehta M, Choi W, Gergis S, Sokoll MD & Adolphson A. Facilitation of endotracheal intubations with divided doses of non-depolarizing neuromuscular drugs. *Anesthesiology* 1985; **62:** 392–395

8. Taboada J, Rupp S & Miller RD. Refining the priming principle for vecuronium during rapid sequence induction of anaesthesia. *Anesthesiology* 1986; **64:** 243–247

9. James MFM, Schenk PA & Vander Veen BW. Priming of pancuronium with magnesium. *Br J Anaesth* 1991; **4:** 247–249

10. Kirkgaard Nielson H, May O, Ravlo MD & Bach V. Priming principle with atracurium. *Acta Anaesth Belg* 1990; **41:** 313–317

11. Brady MM, Mirakhur AD, Clarke RSJ & Gibson FM. Administration of atracurium or vecuronium in divided doses do not accelerate onset. *Anesthesiology* 1987; **67:** A347

12. Ramsey FM, Weeks DB, Morell RC & Gerr P. The priming principle ineffectiveness of atracurium pre treatment. *Anesthesiology* 1987; **67:** A341

13. Donati F, Lahoud J, Walsh CM *et al.* Onset of pancuronium and *d*-tubocurarine blockade with priming. *Can J Anaesth* 1986; **33:** 571–577

14. Pollard BJ. Priming with alcuronium and tubocurarine accelerates the onset of neuromuscular block. *Br J Anaesth* 1989; **63:** 7–11

15. Harrop-Griffiths AW, Grounds RM & Moore M. Intubating conditions following pre induction priming with alcuronium. *Anaesthesia* 1986; **41:** 282–286

16. Van Aken H, Mertes N & Hauss GM. Pretreatment technique for fast intubation with vecuronium: intubation conditions and unwanted effects. *Acta Anaesthesiol Belg* 1986; **37:** 199–201

17. Engbeck J & Viby Morgensen J. Precurarisation – a hazard to the patient? *Acta Anaesthesiol Scand* 1984; **28:** 61–62

18. Haxby EJ, Hood JR, Golpinath RS & Feldman SA. Mivacurium priming intervals. *Br J Anaesth* 1994; **73:** 724

19. Feldman SA. Update on muscle relaxants. *Br J Hosp Med* 1993; **52:** 142–149

20. Epstein RH & Bartkowski RR. Priming v timing. Predictions of a receptor binding model of the neuromuscular junction. *Anesth Analg* 1993; **76:** 597

21. Redai I & Feldman SA. Priming studies with rocuronium and vecuronium. *Eur J Anaesth* 1995; **12:** 11–15

14

Depolarizing neuromuscular block

The paper of Crum-Brown and Fraser[1] in the late 19th century first drew attention to the paralysing properties of some quaternary ammonium salts. In 1948 the neuromuscular blocking action of decamethonium (C_{10}), a bisquaternary salt, was investigated by Barlow and Ing[2] and by Paton and Zaimis.[3] Brown et al.[4] demonstrated that the drug caused an acetyl-choline (ACh)-like depolarization of the postsynaptic membrane, leading to a reduction of the end-plate potential and to neuromuscular block. In 1953 Jenerick and Gerard[5] demonstrated that neuromuscular trans-mission in a single muscle fibre preparation was blocked if the resting membrane potential was reduced from -90 to -57 mV. The observation of Brown et al.[4] and del Castillo and Katz[6] that it was possible to approach this degree of depolarization briefly by exposure to C_{10} seemed to prove that the block produced by the drug was due to a partial post-synaptic depolarization which was itself insufficient to trigger an action potential. Initially there was a reluctance to accept the concept that neuro-muscular block could be caused by depolarization as the result of drug action, although cathodal block, the physiological equivalent of depolar-ization, had been demonstrated for many years.

Gissen and Nastuk[7] also demonstrated partial depolarization of the postsynaptic membrane with suxamethonium, but their experiments failed to achieve a sufficient degree of end-plate depolarization to explain neuro-muscular block. Increasing the suxamethonium concentration further reduced the degree of depolarization. However, they did demonstrate a depolarization to -60 mV with C_{10} although, like suxamethonium, increas-ing the C_{10} concentration further resulted in a reduction in this effect (Fig. 14.1). With the advent of patch-clamping the channel-opening effect associated with a reduction in the transmembrane potential by C_{10} and suberyldicholine has been clearly demonstrated at the receptor level.[8] It is now completely accepted that depolarizing drugs do increase the channel open time either by delaying closure or increasing the frequency of channel opening and thus produce a membrane current flux which produces some degree of postsynaptic depolarization.

It was on the basis of these observations that it has become widely accepted that the mechanism of the block produced by suxamethonium and C_{10} is due to a lowering of the postsynaptic transmembrane potential

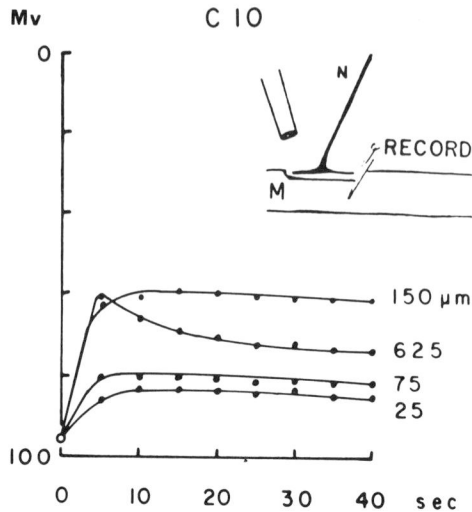

Fig. 14.1 Increasing the concentration of C_{10} to 150 μm produced 40 mV depolarization (to -60 mV) but further increases in drug concentration caused less effect. After Gissen and Nastuk.[7]

to a level that produces neuromuscular block. As a result they have been classified as depolarizing in nature.

However, various observations demand that this view be questioned:

1 Many years ago Zaimis demonstrated that C_{10} administered to a starling that flew into her laboratory caused sustained contraction of its neck muscles, followed by relaxation. Zaimis studied the response to depolarizing drugs on avian cervical muscle (a multiply innervated muscle). They recorded a dual response of contracture followed by relaxation.[9] This effect of initial contraction followed by relaxation in the presence of the same concentration of C_{10} was later described in newborn human intercostal muscle, a focally innervated structure. The cause of the contracture produced by C_{10} has never been explained, as it does not occur following close intra-arterial injection of ACh in normal muscles.[10] However, it is similar to that seen in denervated, focally innervated mammalian muscle exposed to ACh. If C_{10} is injected intra-arterially into a cat tibialis anterior muscle preparation, it causes only a brief ACh-like contraction rather than paralysis as it is washed through the preparation.[11] This suggests that, although it is not uncommon to observe a small (<10%) increase in twitch tension following the injection of C_{10} in humans, the normal blockade of neuromuscular transmission requires either a longer or larger exposure to the drug.

2 Thesleff[12] demonstrated that the initial depolarization of the postsynaptic membrane is short-lived and that even after the membrane potential returns to resting levels the muscle remains paralysed. He attributed the prolonged paralysis to 'desensitization' which outlasts the brief period of depolarization.

3 Riker,[13,14] Standaert and Adams[15] and Galindo[16] have all suggested that ACh and depolarizing drugs have a presynaptic effect. These drugs have

all been demonstrated to cause an initial increase in twitch response, to produce antidromic firing in motor nerves, repetitive afterdischarge following motor nerve stimulation and reduced transmitter release after prolonged exposure – all these events are explicable on the basis of a presynaptic rather than a postsynaptic process.

4 When C_{10} was first introduced and tested on 3 volunteers (the volunteers included Paton and Zaimis), it was demonstrated that C_5 partially antagonized its effect[17] (Fig. 14.2). At the time Paton postulated competitive

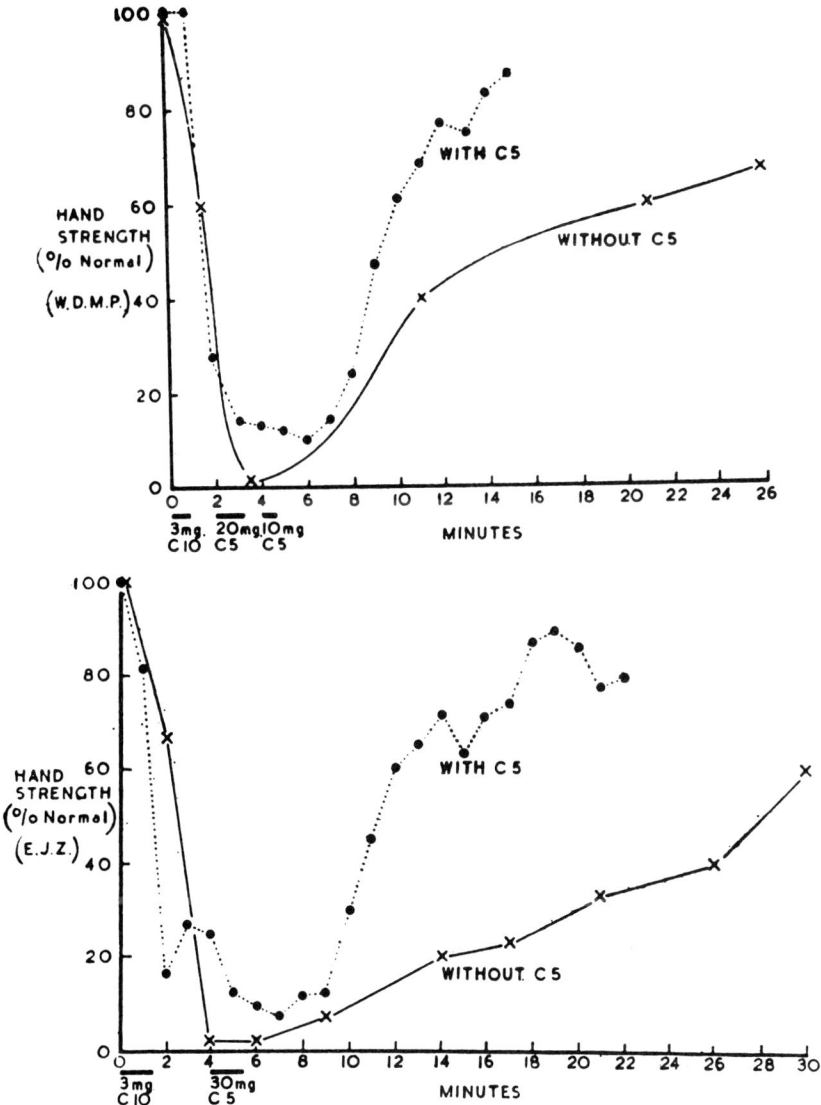

Fig. 14.2 From the original paper on the action of C_{10} in humans.[17] Organe *et al.* demonstrated that C_5 antagonized the block produced by C_{10}. (Note volunteer in upper trace is Paton and in the lower trace Zaimis.)

antagonism resulting from the two similar drugs competing for the same receptors. Ginsborg and Stephenson[18] have demonstrated that if two drugs act at one receptor, the drug having the higher affinity produces the predominant effect. We now know that C_5 acts principally at presynaptic receptors unless given in very large doses (larger than that used by Organe et al.)[17] and, like C_6, produces train-of-four (TOF) and tetanic fade at doses that have little effect on the twitch response. C_5 and C_6 only produce effects on the twitch response with doses far in excess of those required to produce muscarinic ganglionic block and TOF fade. It is probable, therefore, that the reversal of C_{10} action by C_5 is due to competition which occurs at a common presynaptic receptor site and not, as originally believed, at the post-synaptic cholinoceptor.

We have investigated the competition between C_6 and C_{10} in the phrenic nerve diaphragm preparation of rats. We have pretreated the preparation with a dose of C_6 that causes greater than 70% fade of the T_4/T_1 ratio and is associated with less than 10% depression of T_1. As a result of this pretreatment with C_6, there is an approximately 10-fold increase in the ED_{50} dose requirement for C_{10}. This effect has been demonstrated using 50% isobols of C_6 and C_{10}. The resulting isobologram demonstrates marked antagonism of C_{10} by low doses of C_6 (Fig. 14.3).[19]

5 It has been demonstrated that large (1.5 mg/kg) doses of suxamethonium antagonize partial non-depolarizing block,[20,21] i.e. they compete with one another for the same receptor sites (Fig. 14.4). It has also been found that pretreatment with a non-depolarizing drug such as vecuronium causes resistance to subsequent depolarizing drugs (i.e. a shift to the right of the log dose–response curves), indicating antagonism (Fig. 14.5).[22] However, in spite of this evidence of competition between agonist and antagonist drug, pretreatment with C_{10} (and with suxamethonium) reduces the dose requirements of a subsequent non-depolarizing drug. Following recovery from C_{10} block, this results in a shift to the left of the log dose–response curve of vecuronium and a sevenfold reduction in the dose of vecuronium required to produce

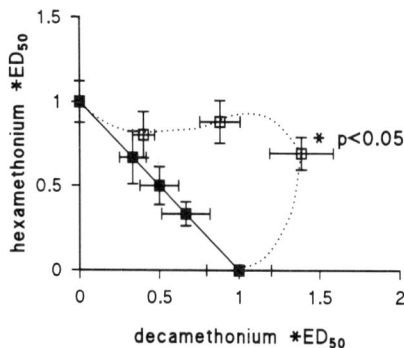

Fig. 14.3 Isobologram of C_6 and C_{10} demonstrating strong antagonism of C_{10} in a preparation treated with C_6. From Redai et al.,[19] with permission.

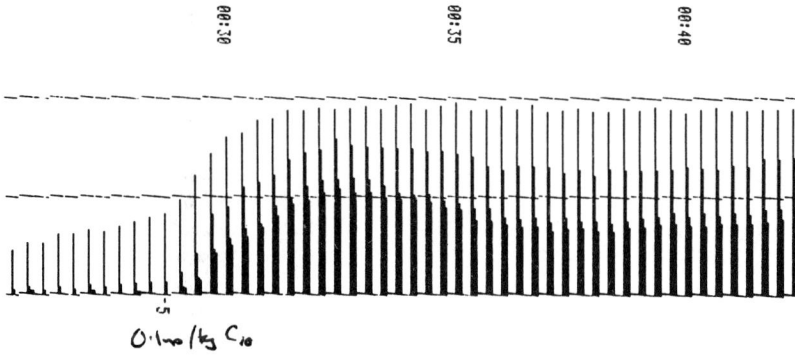

Fig. 14.4 Brief antagonism of tubocurare block by C_{10}. 0.1 mg C_{10} given at '5'.

90% block (Fig. 14.6).[23] Although the antagonism of the two drugs is readily understood as an interaction at the same receptor, it is impossible to explain the apparent synergism resulting from pretreatment with C_{10} on the basis of both drugs competing for the same receptor. Some other mechanism must come into play in addition to the known effect of competition at the postsynaptic receptor.

Although the competition between the ACh and antagonist drug would explain the reversal of non-depolarizing block produced by suxamethonium and the resistance to suxamethonium following non-depolarizing block, it requires an additional action of the drug to explain the synergism. The most likely mechanism would involve the C_{10} (or suxamethonium) acting in a manner that would cause a reduction in the ACh production during the recovery from its blocking effect, thus markedly enhancing the effect of the subsequent administration of vecuronium. It is tempting to suggest that this is the result of the action of the drug at a different site such as a presynaptic receptor rather than changing its role at the same receptor.

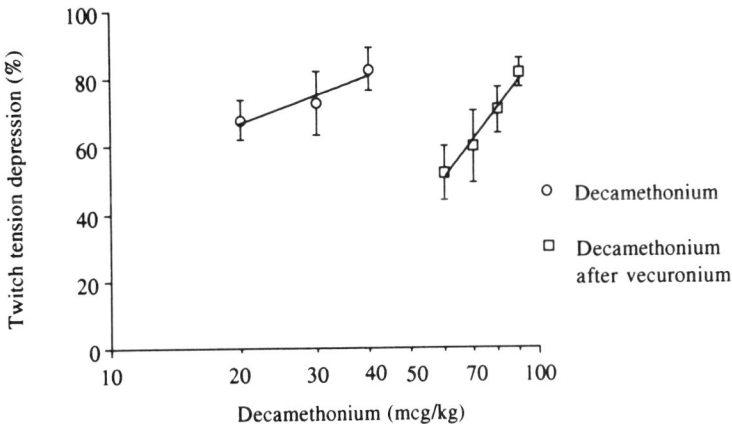

Fig. 14.5 Shift of log dose–response to C_{10} to the right after recovery from vecuronium block, indicating antagonism. Feldman and Fauvel.[23]

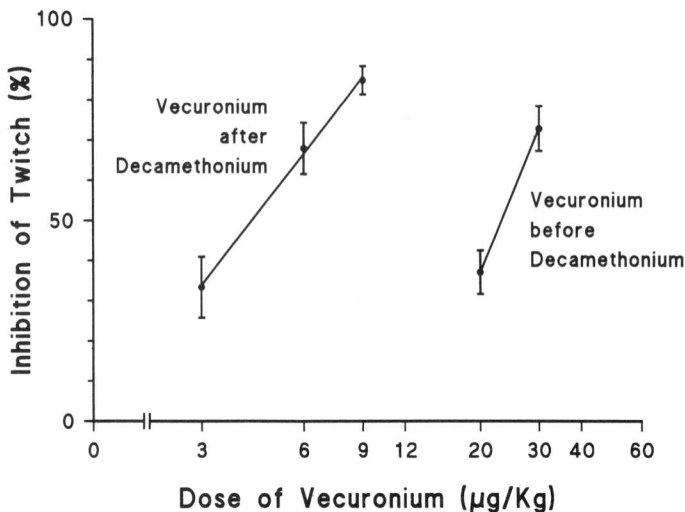

Fig. 14.6 Shift of log dose–response to vecuronium to the left after recovery from C_{10}, indicating synergism.

6 Probably the most convincing evidence of an action of depolarizing drugs at a separate, probably presynaptic receptor, comes from the demonstration that prior treatment with a small dose of non-depolarizing drug, such as that used to prevent muscle fasciculations, affects the rate of onset of suxamethonium block and produces TOF fade. This common observation has previously gone unremarked. It was investigated in some detail using vecuronium together with suxamethonium[24] and more recently by administering two different small doses of tubocurare 10 s before 1 mg/kg suxamethonium (Fig. 14.7).[25] The reason for using the two doses of antagonist drug was to demonstrate that the block produced following the suxamethonium was indeed agonist in nature – less block occurred with higher concentrations of tubocurare.

It was observed in these experiments that the onset of suxamethonium block was slowed by prior treatment with tubocurare and the onset and recovery were associated with TOF fade. This clearly demonstrates that the tubocurare administered 10 s before the suxamethonium was present at the receptor site at the time the suxamethonium arrived at the site and at the time the suxamethonium was starting to act (it is apparent therefore that the slower onset of tubocurare block, relative to suxamethonium, is not due to inability to reach the receptor site as rapidly as suxamethonium but that it must be the result of a slower onset of effect at the receptor). However, the most interesting observation is the occurrence of TOF fade during the subsequent agonist block. If it is accepted that the TOF fade is due to the tubocurare acting at a presynaptic nicotinic receptor site reducing ACh output so that ACh output at $T_1 > T_2 > T_3 > T_4$, i.e. T_4 stimulation produces less ACh (agonist) than T_4, then it is impossible to explain why, when the maximum agonist concentration is present (suxamethonium + ACh), i.e. at the first twitch (T_1), the block observed is less than at T_4. At T_4 there should be the

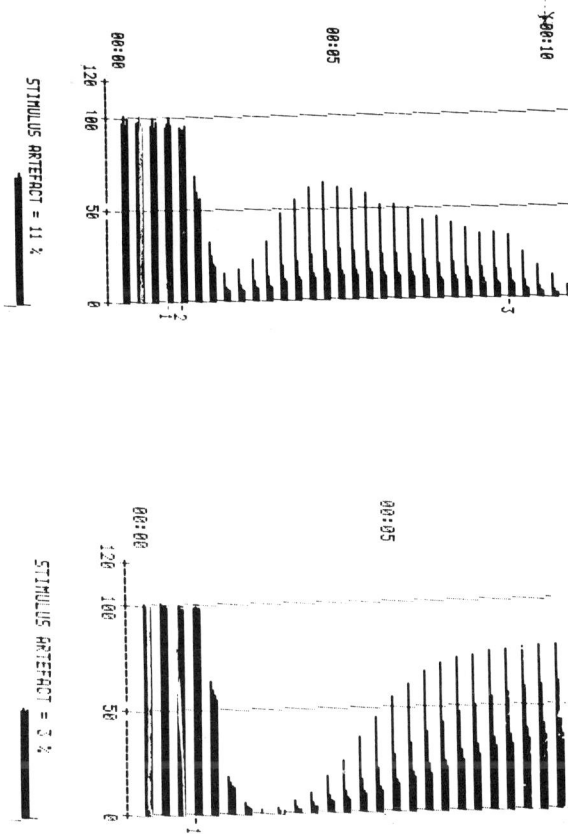

Fig. 14.7 Effect of prior administration of tubocurare (upper trace 0.25 mg/kg, lower trace 0.125 mg/kg) 10 s before administration of 1 mg/kg suxamethonium. Note that there is more block with a lower dose of tubocurare, indicating agonist block, slower onset of suxamethonium block (60–80 s) and train of four fade during onset and recovery. In the upper trace a slower onset of tubocurare block (3) was recorded.

lowest receptor concentration of ACh to act synergistically with the suxamethonium and hence the least block resulting in the greatest twitch response, whereas T_4 is the smallest response observed. TOF fade can be explained during antagonist block on the basis of diminishing ACh output, but this does not explain its occurrence during an agonist block. Instead, one should observe a TOF enhancement during an agonist block if it is caused by a progressive fall in ACh production from T_1 to T_4 and that the site of block is at the postsynaptic receptor site. If one accepts TOF as a presynaptic event then its presence during suxamethonium block must indicate that at least some of the usual activity of suxamethonium is due to an action at the presynaptic receptor which, in these circumstances, has already been partially blocked by the tubocurare. It follows that the usual action of C_{10} at this site would be to cause ACh release, adding to its postsynaptic depolarizing action, an activity reduced by pretreatment with tubocurare.

We therefore have strong but circumstantial evidence, that drugs such as suxamethonium and C_{10} act at presynaptic sites in addition to their proven ability to produce modest degrees of postsynaptic depolarization. This evidence was presented in a review by Feldman and Hood.[26] A presynaptic site of action would also explain why neither C_{10} nor suxamethonium alone has been demonstrated to produce the level of postsynaptic depolarization necessary to cause a depolarizing block. It would explain the observations of Thesleff[12,27] and Katz and Thesleff[28] that the postsynaptic depolarization does not last as long as the neuromuscular block.

By analogy with other drugs that act presynaptically, such as edrophonium and neostigmine, it would be expected that the initial response would be to stimulate ACh discharge followed by a presynaptic block, either due to the ill-understood mechanism termed desensitization,[28] or due to a rundown of presynaptic ACh stores. Such an action would explain the effect seen by Zaimis and coworkers in avian muscle – a tonic contraction followed by flaccid paralysis. It would also help us understand the mechanism by which phase II block develops. However, it would not rule out the possibility that phase II block was caused by a separate postsynaptic curare-like action of the drug.

It is difficult to envisage that the evidence suggesting a presynaptic site of action of suxamethonium is of only minor importance in the production of its clinical effect. It is probable that a large part of the block produced by these drugs is due to presynaptic stimulation followed by desensitization or rundown of ACh stores.

A presynaptic site of action would help explain the antidromic motor nerve discharge that occurs in animals following suxamethonium administration and the hypertensive response caused by ganglionic stimulation that was reported by Bovet in his early animal experiments with suxamethonium. Such an action would also explain the repetitive afterdischarge found following stimulation of a motor nerve in the presence of depolarizing drug.[15] It is possible also that the fasciculations seen with suxamethonium are associated with ACh released as a consequence of the presynaptic effect on the n_{rep} receptors by the drug. A presynaptic site of action would also explain the reduced effect of suxamethonium after magnesium.[29] It is well-recognized that magnesium reduces ACh release following motor nerve stimulation and it is anticipated that it would also reduce the effectiveness of suxamethonium if it acted through a similar mechanism.

It seems probable that drugs such as C_{10} and suxamethonium act at both presynaptic n_{mob} and n_{rep} receptors and at postsynaptic sites and the depolarizing block is due in part to the ACh released presynaptically. It is implicit that depolarizing drugs do not act in the same way as the non-depolarizing agents. Whereas a non-depolarizing drug is taken up in the biophase to form a reservoir, the activity of depolarizing drugs parallels their plasma and ECF concentration. Thus, a depolarizing drug such as suxamethonium will cease to act once its plasma level has been reduced to subclinical levels by hydrolysis, as the drug will be washed out of the synapse, whereas mivacurium, which is hydrolysed at a similar rate to suxamethonium, produces a block that continues long after its plasma level has fallen to subclinical levels due to a residual reservoir of drug in the biophase binding sites. Because of this difference recovery from depolarizing block is affected by changes in blood flow and plasma concentration whereas non-depolarizing block is only indirectly affected by the plasma concentration and its effect prolonged only if the blood flow falls to levels likely to produce tissue hypoxia.[30,31]

It is likely that a presynaptic nicotinic receptor would be a far simpler pentameric structure than that at the postsynaptic membrane; it follows therefore that binding to biophase acceptor sites is less likely to occur. If we accept that depolarizing neuromuscular blocking drugs react at the presynaptic site by a simple physical process which causes their onset and offset to be governed by diffusion along concentration gradients, whereas non-depolarizing agents undergo binding and dissociation in the biophase, we have a clearer understanding of why the nature of the block produced by depolarizing drugs differs from that produced by non-depolarizing agents. It offers an explanation of why the block occurs rapidly and recovers more quickly than that caused by non-depolarizing agents and why recovery from a depolarizing drug such as C_{10} is far quicker in the isolated arm than that for vecuronium, a drug with a similar duration of clinical block (Fig. 14.8).

Further confirmation of the fundamental difference in the drug receptor reaction comes from studies on the effects of hypothermia on the onset and offset of the two types of block. We have demonstrated that a 4–5°C drop in skin temperature markedly affects the rate of both onset and offset of non-depolarizing neuromuscular block with a Q_{10} of >2.8, whilst it has little effect on the onset and offset of C_{10} block (Q_{10} of <1.3). Hill[32] postulated that a physical process such as diffusion would be little affected by temperature ($Q_{10} < 1.4$), whereas a chemical or molecular binding–unbinding process involving a change in entropy would have a $Q_{10} > 2.4$. Our experiments suggest that the reaction between C_{10} and the receptor is a physical process, whereas it is an energy-sensitive binding–unbinding mechanism that controls the onset and offset of non-depolarizing drugs.[33,34] This difference would explain why there is no increase in C_{10} block in the isolated arm following release of the tourniquet at 50% block (see Chapter 6).

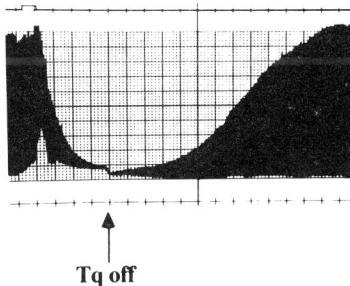

Tq off

Fig. 14.8 In the isolated arm the recovery index for C_{10} is 3 min. Following systemic injection, its duration of action is 20–40 min. Tq = Tourniquet.

If depolarizing drugs have a major presynaptic component to their effect it is possible that it is this site of action that produces the phase II effect. It is well-recognized that drugs such as neostigmine can induce an initial presynaptic stimulation, followed by desensitization. It would seem reasonable to suggest that C_{10} and suxamethonium will have a similar action. However, there remains a significant body of evidence to suggest that a curare-like postsynaptic block may occur and that postsynaptic events such as desensitization may contribute to the development of phase II block. The present evidence is inconclusive but it is evident that phase II block starts to develop soon after the drug is administered and its occurrence is time- rather than dose-dependent[35] (Fig. 14.9). Whatever the cause of phase II block, one has to accept the ability of neostigmine and edrophonium to reverse it. Assuming that the reversal is not due to the anticholinesterase itself, but to the increased survival time of ACh molecules, then it is difficult to explain why ACh should reverse the block, or make good the deficiency caused by the phase II block whilst further agonist drug (either suxamethonium or C_{10}) makes it worse (Fig. 14.10). This effect is difficult to accommodate in terms of a postsynaptic desensitization.

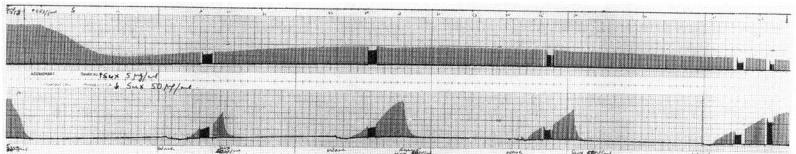

Fig. 14.9 Administration of suxamethonium to two rat phrenic nerve hemidiaphragms over time. Upper trace: 5 μg/ml; lower trace 50 μg/ml (washout every 15 min to test train of four). Note the similar rate of development of tetanic fade in both traces. After Gupta et al.[35]

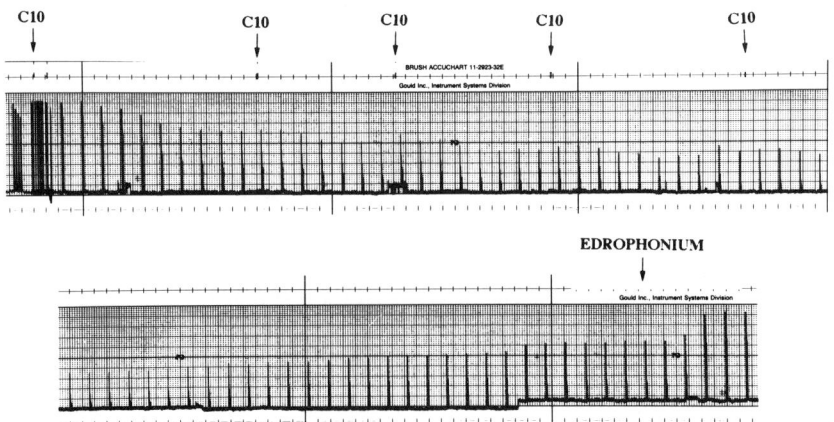

Fig. 14.10 Repeated injections of C_{10} cause increased train-of-four fade and T_1 block. Edrophonium 10 mg reverses T_1 depression and train-of-four fade.

A further observation that is most easily explained in terms of a pre-synaptic action of C_{10} is the finding that there is a positive correlation between the ED_{50} dose of C_{10} and the T_4/T_1 ratio of the TOF, no matter how the TOF fade was produced. Figure 14.11 shows this relationship in a series of patients; in some of these patients the fade resulted from prior C_{10} administration and in others it occurred after recovery of T_1 following vecuronium.

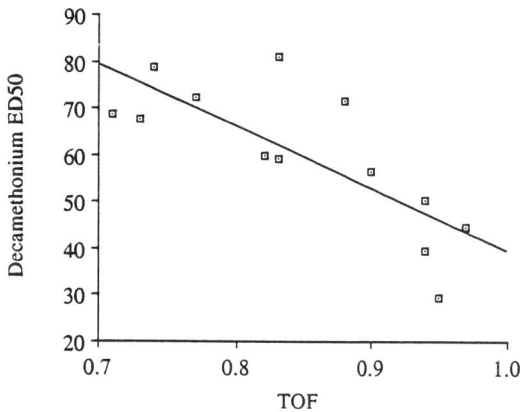

Fig. 14.11 Inverse relationship between train of four (TOF) present (irrespective of how it is produced) and ED_{50} for C_{10}.

Conclusions

Whilst one can explain most, if not all, the events observed with depolarizing drugs in terms of an initial stimulation followed by block of presynaptic receptors, one cannot ignore the undoubted postsynaptic action of these drugs.[35] On balance, it is probable that, like other bisquaternary compounds, they act at both pre- and postsynaptic sites.

References

1. Crum-Brown A & Fraser TR. On the connection between chemical constitution and physiological action. *Trans R Soc Edin* 1868; **25:** 151–158
2. Barlow BB & Ing HR. Curare-like action of polymethylene bisquaternary ammonium salts. *Nature* 1948; **161:** 718
3. Paton WDM & Zaimis EJ. Curare like action of the polymethylene bisquaternary ammonium salts. *Nature* 1948; **161:** 719
4. Brown GL, Paton WDM & Dias VM. The depression of the demarcation potential of the cat's tibialis by α bistrimethlyammonium decane diiodide. *J Physiol* 1949; **109:** 15p
5. Jenerick HP & Gerrard RW. Membrane potential and threshold of single muscle fibre. *J Cell Comp Physiol* 1953; **42:** 79–83
6. del Castillo J & Katz B. Interaction at end plate receptors between different choline derivatives. *Proc R Soc Lond* 1956; **146:** 369–372

7. Gissen AJ & Nastuk WL. Succinylcholine and decamethonium comparison of depolarization and desensitization. *Anesthesiology* 1970; **33:** 611–615

8. Colquhoun D & Sackmann B. Fluctuations in the microsecond time range of the current through a single acetylcholine receptor ion channel. *Nature* 1981; **294:** 646–466

9. Zaimis EJ. Motor end plate differences as a determining factor in the mode of action of neuromuscular blocking substances. *J Physiol* 1953; **22:** 238–251

10. Sabawala PB. (1970) Response of newborn human intercostal muscle to muscle relaxants. In: *Progress in Anaesthesiology. Proceedings of the World Congress of Anaesthesiologists.* Holland: Excerpta Medica

11. Zaimis EJ & Head S. (1976) Depolarizing neuromuscular blocking drugs. In: *Neuromuscular Junction.* Zaimis E (ed.). *Handbook of Experimental Pharmacology.* Berlin: Springer-Verlag. pp. 365–419

12. Thesleff S. The mode of neuromuscular block caused by acetylcholine, decamethonium and succinylcholine on neuromuscular transmission in the rat. *Acta Physiol Scand* 1955; **34:** 386–392

13. Riker WF. Actions of aceylcholine mammalian nerve terminal. *J Pharmacol Exp Ther* 1966; **152:** 397–416

14. Riker WF. (1975) Prejunctional effects of neuromuscular facilitating drugs. In: *Muscle Relaxants.* Katz RL (ed.). North Holland, pp. 59–102

15. Standaert FG & Adams JE. The actions of succinylcholine on mammalian nerve terminals. *J Pharmacol Exp Ther* 1965; **149:** 113–123

16. Galindo A. Depolarizing neuromuscular block. *J Pharmacol Exp Ther* 1971; **178:** 339–346

17. Organe GSW, Paton WDM & Zaimis EJ. Preliminary trials of bistrimethylammonium decane and pentene diodide (C_{10} and C_5) in man. *Lancet* 1949; **1:** 21–25

18. Ginsborg BL & Stephenson RP. On the simultaneous action of two competitive antagonists. *Br J Pharmacol* 1974; **51:** 287–300

19. Redai I, Richards K, England AJ & Feldman SA. Isobolographic analysis of the interaction between hexamethonium and decamethonium. *Anesth Analg* 1995; (in press)

20. Young RB. Suxamethonium for peritoneal closure. *Anaesthesia* 1979; **34:** 716–718

21. Buzello W, Krieg N, Khuls E & Schlickwewi A. Modification of pancuronium induced non-depolarizing neuromuscular block by succinylcholine in anaesthetised humans. *Anesthesiology* 1983; **59:** 573–576

22. Campkin NTA, Hood JR & Feldman SA. Resistance to decamethonium neuromuscular block after prior administration of vecuronium. *Anesth Analg* 1993; **77:** 78–80

23. Feldman SA & Fauvel N. Potentiation and antagonism of vecuronium by decamethonium. *Anesth Analg* 1993; **76:** 631–634

24. Feldman SA, Fauvel NJ & Harrop-Griffiths W. (1990) The onset of neuromuscular blockade. In: *Neuromuscular Blocking Agents, Past, Present and Future.* Bowman WC, Denissen PAF & Feldman SA (eds). Holland: Excerpta Medica, pp. 44–52

25. Hood JR, Campkin NTA & Feldman SA. Curare modification of suxamethonium blockade. *Anaesthesia* 1994; **49:** 682–685

26. Feldman SA & Hood JR. Depolarizing neuromuscular block. A presynaptic site of action? *Acta Anesthesiol Scand* 1994; **38:** 535–541

27. Thesleff S. Motor endplate desentization by repetitive nerve stimulation. *J Physiol* 1959; **148:** 659–664

28. Katz B & Thesleff S. A study of 'desensitization' produced by acetylcholine at the motor end plate. *J Physiol* 1957; **138:** 63–69

29. Tsai SK, Huang SW & Lec TY. Neuromuscular interactions between suxamethonium and magnesium sulphate in the cat. *Br J Anaesth* 1994; **72:** 674–678

30. Feldman SA, Fauvel NJ & Strickland D. (1990) The offset of neuromuscular blockade. In: *Neuromuscular Blocking Agents, Past, Present and Future.* Bowman WC, Denissen PAF & Feldman SA (eds). Holland: Excerpta Medica, pp. 52–60

31. Feldman SA. Biophase binding: its effect on recovery from non-depolarizing neuromuscular block. *Anaesth Pharmacol Rev* 1993; **1:** 81–87

32. Hill AV. *J Physiol Lond* 1909; **39:** 361–373
33. England AJ, Richards K, Redai I, Wu X & Feldman SA. The influence of cold on the recovery index of vercuronium and decamethonium in man. *Br J Anaesth* 1995; **74:** 473P
34. England AJ. The effect of moderate hypothermia on recovery from neuromuscular block induced with C_{10}, vecuronium and atracurium in man. *Anaesthesia* 1996 (to be published)
35. Gupta VJ, Fauvel NJ & Feldman SA. Investigation of fade in suxamethonium induced phase II block in the isolated rate diaphragm. *Br J Anaesth* 1992; **68:** 354P

15

Hypothermia and neuromuscular block

In 1951 Homes et al.[1] suggested that cold antagonized the neuromuscular block produced by curare. Their conclusion came from the observation that cold produced a reduction in the degree of curare-induced neuromuscular block in the rat phrenic nerve diaphragm preparation. This action appeared to be confirmed by the findings of Canard and Zaimis[2] and Zaimis et al.[3] in humans. Zaimis and her colleagues studied the effect of minor degrees of surface cooling upon the action of curare and decamethonium (C_{10}) using a leg calliper device into which strain gauges had been incorporated, allowing the tension developed following dorsiflexion of the foot to be measured in response to stimulation of the lateral popliteal nerve as it crosses the head of the fibula. They recorded four occasions in which there was an increase in muscle contraction following partial block by curare out of six experiments; they also noted potentiation of the partial block produced by C_{10}.[3] As a result of these experiments it was accepted that cold potentiated depolarizing block and antagonized non-depolarizing block. Indeed, Paton[4] suggested that a possible cause of the failure to reverse curare easily at the end of an operation might be associated with rewarming recurarization. This assumption became generally accepted and the company literature which accompanied pancuronium when it was introduced warned against the increased requirements during hypothermia and the risk of rewarming recurarization. This anticurare effect was also reported by Buzello et al.[5] using the compound electromyogram (EMG) as a measure of muscle response to indirect stimulation.

In 1970–71 hypothermia was commonly used during cardiac surgery and at Westminster Hospital the technique of profound hypothermia was pioneered using an extracorporeal blood-cooling system. It was soon obvious that the requirements of non-depolarizing drugs such as tubocurare were, in fact, reduced at lowered muscle temperatures. In 1973 the effect of cooling that was sufficient to produce a fall in forearm muscle temperature of 4–5°C was studied. The adductor pollicis twitch response to stimulation of the ulnar nerve was measured in 4 children in the absence of any muscle relaxant (Fig. 15.1).[6] It showed an approximately 50% fall in the indirectly elicited twitch response with a 5°C fall in muscle temperature. It was difficult to reconcile this observation with the antagonism to curare block previously reported. These initial observations in patients were followed by a series of 10 experiments in dogs presented in 1975,[7] in

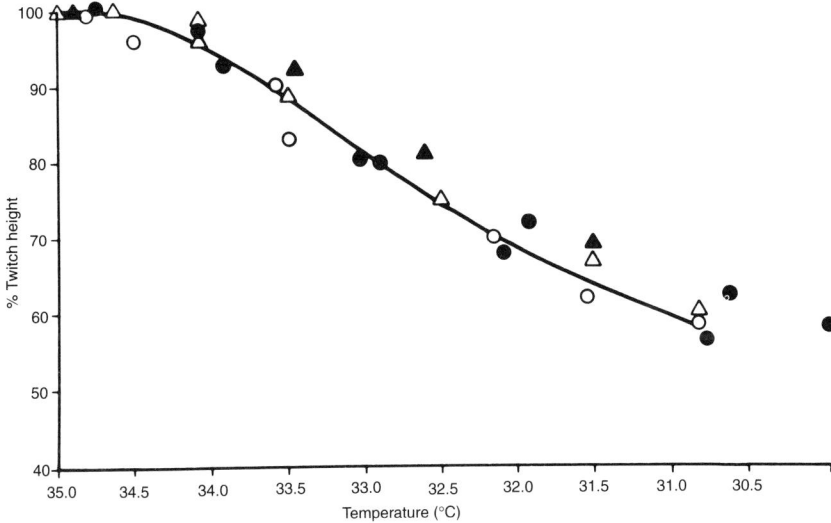

Fig. 15.1 The decrease in adductor pollicis twitch response to indirect stimulation in 4 children during profound hypothermia. Muscle temperature decreased approximately 5°C.

which an extracorporeal cooling circuit allowed constant perfusion of one hind leg with cold blood. These experiments demonstrated that in the dog there was a similar 50–60% fall in the indirectly elicited twitch response over a 5–7°C fall of temperature, whilst direct stimulation of the muscle showed much less depression (Figs 15.2 and 15.3). Interestingly, it was found that further cooling only produced a modest further fall in the indirect twitch response. It was also observed that edrophonium largely corrected this cold-induced neuromuscular block. It was as if each dog reduced the neuromuscular response by a set amount at a temperature that was specific for that animal.

About this time, Foldes et al.[8] described their results in the phrenic nerve diaphragm preparation of rats; this contradicted the findings of Holmes et al.[1] by demonstrating the potentiation of the blocking effects of non-depolarizing drugs by cold. These results were confirmed in cats by Miller et al.[9] and by Ham et al.[10]

Why then were the initial reports of the Los Angeles pharmacologists and of Zaimis's group in London so misleading? After all these years, we can only speculate. In a recent series of rat phrenic nerve diaphragm experiments carried out in our laboratories by Fauvel (personal communication), the unpredictability of the response of this preparation was demonstrated. In very carefully controlled experiments he demonstrated that the usual response of this particular preparation to cooling was to increase both the directly and indirectly elicited twitch response by 20–40%. However, a minority of diaphragms demonstrated the typical reduction in the indirectly elicited twitch we had found in dogs and in children. As a result of the increase in muscle response produced by cold, there can be an apparent antagonism to tubocurare block. It is probable that in the Zaimis experiments the problem was caused by the position of

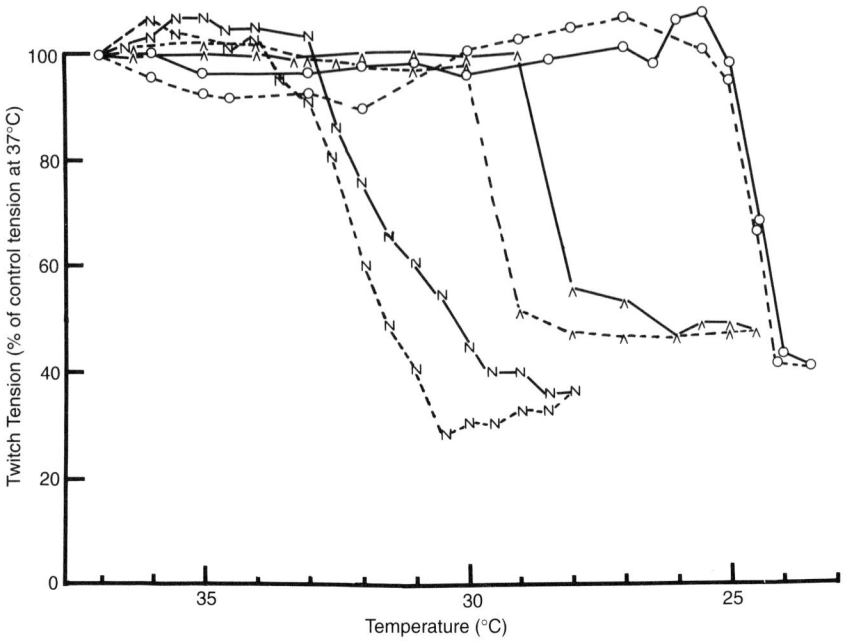

Fig. 15.2 Effect of temperature on indirectly elicited soleus twitch response in 3 dogs during extracorporeal cooling and rewarming of muscles of the hind limb. Note the hysteresis effect on rewarming. All the dogs studied showed a fall in twitch response at a particular critical threshold. Dashed line = rewarming.

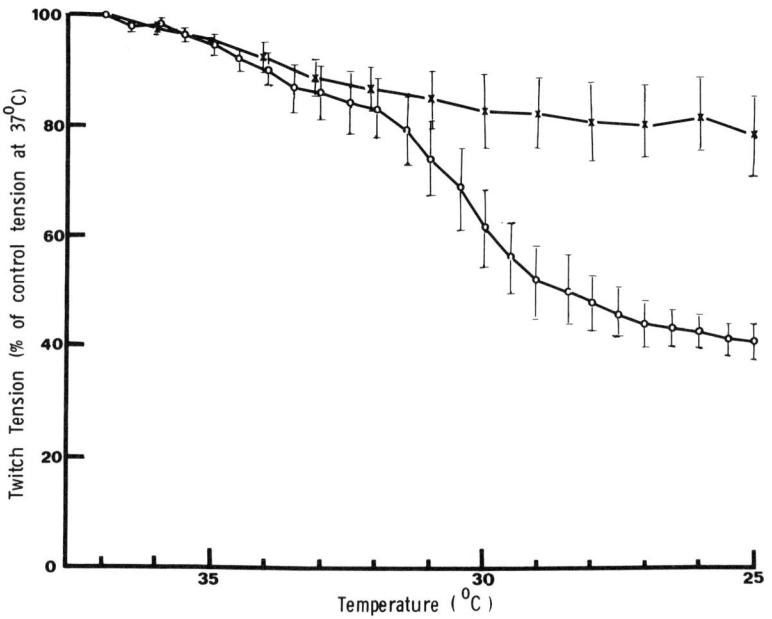

Fig. 15.3 Mean decrease in soleus twitch response to direct (x) and indirect (○) stimulation during hypothermia in dog soleus muscle.

the stimulating electrode. In further experiments we have observed that, unless the lateral popliteal nerve is accurately localized, it is easy to stimulate the muscle of tibialis anterior, causing a direct muscle twitch rather than an indirect one. Indeed, it is common to stimulate both and to obtain a double response using the Zaimis leg calliper.

In an effort to unravel the confusion and to understand why the early workers using the rat phrenic nerve diaphragm preparation reported antagonism to curare during hypothermia, we have studied the response to cold in the rat and the guinea-pig phrenic nerve diaphragm and also the effect of cold upon non-depolarizing neuromuscular block in these animals. England[11] has confirmed Fauvel's observation that cold usually increases both direct and indirect muscle response in the rat (Fig. 15.4). However, in the guinea-pig, whilst cold modestly increases the muscle response initially to both direct and indirect stimulation, at lower temperatures, within a 10°C temperature range, it decreases the response to indirect stimulation (Fig. 15.5a). This effect is accompanied by the development of

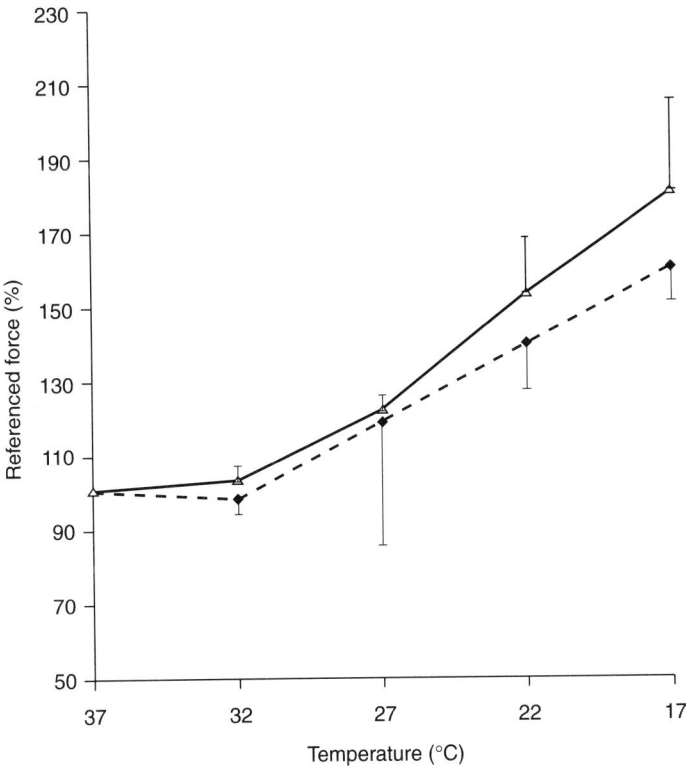

Fig. 15.4 Effect of cooling on the direct and indirect elicited twitch response in the rat diaphragm. Solid lines = response of direct stimulation; dashed lines = response to indirect stimulation. After England.[11]

marked train-of-four (TOF) fade (Fig. 15.5b). In this, the guinea pig diaphragm approaches the response found in the dog. The dog demonstrates
a small decline in direct muscle response with cold but a marked fall in
the response to indirect stimulation. It seems that the nearer the animal
species studied is phylogenetically to a hibernating or poikilothermic
genus the less likely is cold to depress neuromuscular conduction. In
higher animals and humans cold depresses neuromuscular conduction to a
much greater extent than its effect on muscle contraction.

It is now accepted that, contrary to what had been believed until 1972,
cold potentiates non-depolarizing block and reduces the indirectly elicited
twitch response in humans. We have also observed a modest reduction in
the block produced by C_{10} when the temperature of an arm is reduced
from 32 to 27°C.

Mechanism of action of cold

Cold may affect neuromuscular conduction and hence the action of the
muscle relaxants in one of several ways, or by a combination of them:

1 It may affect motor nerve conduction.[12]
2 It may affect the synthesis, storage or mobilization of acetylcholine
  (ACh).[13]

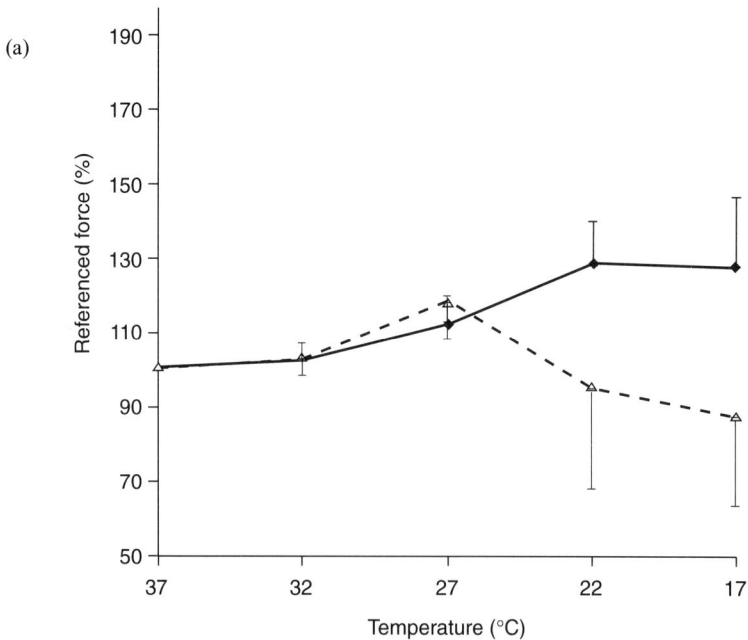

(a)

Fig. 15.5 (a) Effect of cooling on the direct and indirect elicited twitch response in the
guinea-pig diaphragm. Solid line = response of direct stimulation; dashed line = response to
indirect stimulation. After England.[11]

(b)

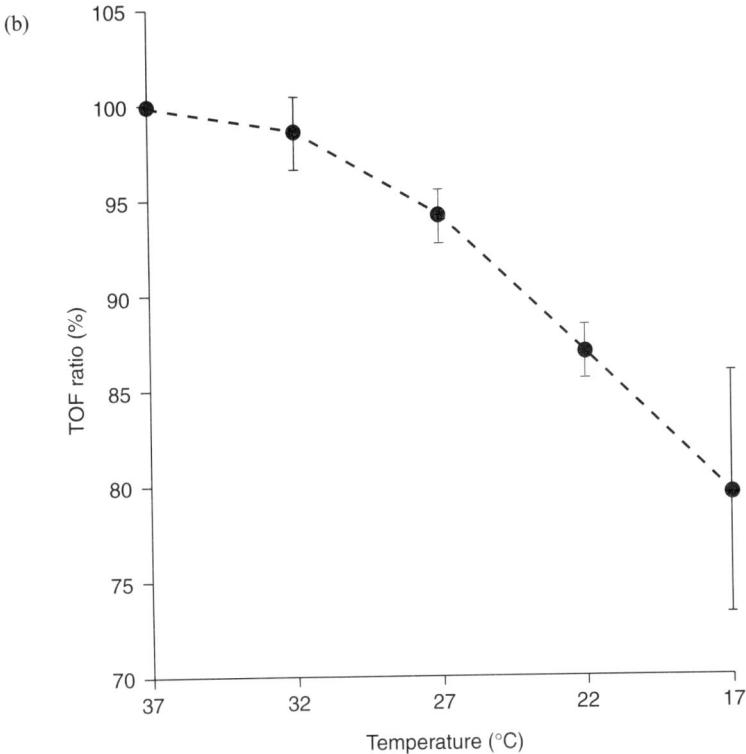

Fig. 15.5 (b) Effect of cooling on train-of-four (TOF) ratio in the indirectly stimulated guinea-pig diaphragm. After England.[11]

3 It may affect ACh release and synaptic transmission.[14,15]
4 It may depress acetylcholinesterase.[24]
5 It may affect muscle contraction.[16,17]
6 It may affect cell membrane repolarization.[18,19]

In addition there is little doubt that cold has a pronounced effect upon the pharmacokinetics of drugs by affecting metabolism and hepatic and renal excretion.[10,20–22]

Cold and nerve conduction

It has been known, since the observations of Lorenté de No, that cold blocked neural conduction. The effect of cold on motor nerve conduction was studied in the squid axon by Hodgkin and Katz,[19] who demonstrated conduction delay at lowered temperature. It is probable that this effect is produced by an action on the K^+ channels at the nodes of Ranvier. The modest temperature changes produced in patients by anaesthesia and surgery are unlikely to cause a clinically detectable effect.

Synthesis, storage and mobilization of acetylcholine

Many parts of the ACh synthesis, storage and mobilization cycle require a transfer of energy, usually through the calmodulin–adenosine triphosphatase (ATPase) mechanism. These mechanisms would be expected to be depressed by hypothermia. Cold affects the transport of choline into the motor nerve. This active carrier transport mechanism has been demonstrated to be temperature-sensitive.[23] The acetylation of choline is an active enzymatic process and is depressed *in vitro* by cold.[13] The 'packaging' of ACh in the vesicles against a concentration gradient is an energy-dependent process and it is anticipated that this would be less effective at lower temperatures. The mobilization of stored ACh vesicles by Ca^{2+} involves calmodulin and ATPase, a process known to be temperature-sensitive. Thus, cooling would be expected to have a cumulative effect from its actions at many sites, which would slow the rate at which readily releasable ACh becomes available and the amount of ACh released by motor nerve activity.[14] This is likely to be overwhelmed by the normal excess ACh released and may only be clinically significant if the amount of ACh released was marginal or in the presence of some presynaptic or postsynaptic block, such as that caused by a non-depolarizing drug. Because of the size of the normal reserve, the effect may not be obvious in the absence of partial neuromuscular block or some predisposing effect.

We have demonstrated a small ($<15\%$) T_4/T_1 fade in volunteers in whom an arm was cooled to produce a 5°C drop in skin temperature and in whom the twitch response was reduced by 10–20% (Fig. 15.6). The suggestion that hypothermia produces at least some of its effect by depressing the ACh production release mechanism is supported by the observation that in children and dogs under hypothermia, in whom the muscle temperature was reduced by 5°C and the indirect twitch response depressed, there was a positive response to edrophonium which produced almost complete restoration of the twitch. It is possible that this may represent a direct

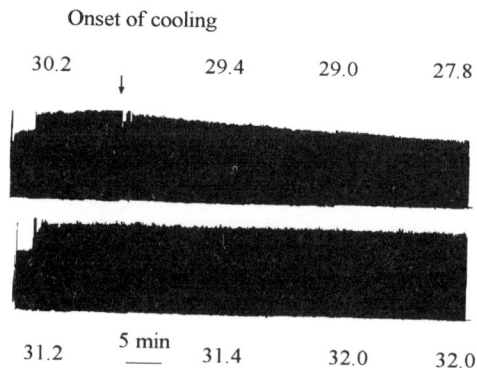

Fig. 15.6 Effect of cooling on the indirectly elicited adductor pollicis twitch of volunteers (lower trace: contralateral control arm). The upper tracing was cooled from 30.2 to 27.8°C; the lower trace was maintained at between 31.2 and 32.0°C.

A stabilization period of 10 min was allowed before cooling.

The trace shows no depression of force of contraction of the control arm and a fall in force of contraction of 20% for a temperature drop of 2.4°C in the cooled arm.

effect of edrophonium presynaptically, but it is tempting to see this as evidence that at least some of the twitch depression caused by cooling is due to depression of the ACh mechanism. An acceptance of this mechanism also helps to explain the increase in the ED_{50} requirements of C_{10} we have observed during hypothermia.[11]

Acetylcholine

The extrusion of the contents of the ACh vesicles at the active zone of the presynaptic membrane requires Ca^{2+} activation of synaptotagmin and synaptophysin. It may be the interference with this mechanism or an increase in the reaction time required to activate the ACh receptors that causes the increased synaptic delay demonstrated by Katz and Miledi under hypothermia.[15] It is unlikely to be due to an effect on diffusion across the synaptic cleft, as this physical process would be much less affected by cooling.

Depression of acetylcholinesterase

In vitro the action of acetylcholinesterase is reduced upon cooling the media.[24] This illustrates the complexity of the picture produced by cold, which is likely to reduce ACh synthesis and release, but at the same time depresses the enzyme that hydrolyses the transmitter so, theoretically, potentiate its action and increases its effectiveness.

Muscle contraction

Moderate cold generally increases muscle contractility.[17,25,26] This is probably the result of delayed closure of Ca^{2+} channels, resulting in an increased influx of Ca^{2+} into sarcoplasmic reticulum and increasing the rate of activation of the actin–myosin reaction. This effect is much more marked in lower animal species. Attempts to use cold to increase muscle response in myotonia and myasthenia have failed to produce an improvement.

Repolarization of cell membranes

Repolarization of cell membranes involves the Na/K pump mechanism which is energy-dependent and sensitive to temperature change. Delayed repolarization would be expected to increase muscle contractility[27] and to potentiate the action of depolarizing drug.[25] Although Zaimis reported the potentiation of C_{10} in humans, we have only observed antagonism to C_{10} in the rat phrenic nerve diaphragm preparation. This effect of cold on repolarization of cell membranes would also be expected to mitigate the effect of reduced ACh release.

It is possible that this site of action of cooling may explain why observations made on the effect of hypothermia using the EMG often differ from those using mechanomyography.[28] It could be anticipated that the effect on the compound voltage change might differ from the mechanical response of cooling due to delayed repolarization of the membrane, causing a greater total electromotive force during the measurement of a compound EMG.

Experimental observations on the effect of cold on neuromuscular conduction and block

The effect of cold on neuromuscular conduction in humans has usually demonstrated a depression of twitch response. Efforts to determine a true Q_{10} for the effect of cold would necessitate monitoring the temperature of the muscle being studied over a 10°C temperature change. This is difficult to justify in patients or volunteers. As a result, the depression of twitch associated with a 5°C drop in core temperature has usually been assessed. This produces about 10–20% depression of T_1, depending upon the method of recording used. In our studies in conscious volunteers we have observed a mean 12% depression of adductor pollicis twitch produced by a 5°C drop in skin temperature (measured over the thenar eminence) caused by surface cooling (Fig. 15.5).

Studies in humans either during cardiac surgery[24] or following continuous drug infusion[22] have usually demonstrated the potentiation of non-depolarizing neuromuscular block associated with a reduced distribution volume for the drug. The importance of the pharmacokinetic element in the potentiation of the action of the non-depolarizing drugs is evident. This effect is less likely to be seen following a small single dose of drug, as cold is unlikely to affect redistribution and the initial rapid decay in the plasma concentration. However, following continuous infusion of drugs that are metabolized in the liver or are excreted by the liver and kidneys – all processes that are depressed by hypothermia – a prolonged action would be anticipated as a result of a reduction in plasma clearance of drug. It will be of interest to observe if this effect also occurs with miva-curium and atracurium as the metabolism by cholinesterase should be depressed to a greater extent than Hofmann degradation.

What is less clear is how much of the effect of hypothermia on the action of the muscle relaxants in humans is due to altered metabolism and excretion and how much is due to the effect of cold at the synapse. Indeed, there is a lack of agreement on the contribution of effects at the neuromuscular junction to the potentation of action observed. In an effort to separate these effects we have performed a series of forearm experiments on both arms of volunteers. In these experiments one forearm was cooled by icepacks whilst the other was kept normothermic. When the skin temperature of the cold arm had been reduced by >5°C both forearms were simultaneously isolated from the circulation by means of tourniquets and 0.3 mg vecuronium in 20 ml of saline was injected intravenously into both isolated forearms. Onset of block was studied by releasing the tourniquet at 20% block and observing the time to achieve 80% block. The amount of block and the time to recover from 20% to 80% twitch height were noted.

It was observed that, although the 4–5.5°C skin differential produced between the cold arm and the control warm arm decreased the twitch response of the cold arm, the effect of the given dose of vecuronium was equipotent in both forearms. Cold did not increase the amount of block produced. However, cold considerably delayed both the onset and recovery of block, thus both the onset and offset were some 75% slower in the cold arm. The calculated Q_{10} of onset and offset of vecuronium block was increased (Fig. 15.7). For onset it was 2.6 ± 1.2 and for offset 2.9 ± 0.88.[29] It is of interest that this is at variance with the findings of Glavinovic et al. using iontophoretic pulses of non-depolarizing drugs and ACh in frog muscle.[30] These workers showed a very modest slowing of T_{on} and T_{off} with a Q_{10} of 1.3 following cooling. This probably reflects the well-documented difference in the effect of cold in hibernating and poikilo-thermic animals compared to higher species.[31] When the double isolated arm experiment was carried out to investigate the effect of hypothermia using C_{10} (0.15 mg in 20 ml saline), the tourniquet had to be released at 80% block in order to achieve sufficient paralysis to measure T_{off} in these experiments. The Q_{10} for the recovery from C_{10} neuromuscular block was 1.2 ± 0.74 (Fig. 15.8).

Since the early work of Hill,[32] the effect of temperature upon the rate of biological process has been used to differentiate between purely physical processes, such as diffusion, and biological processes involving chemical processes such as binding and unbinding at receptors. A Q_{10} of <1.4 strongly suggested a physical process, whereas a $Q_{10} > 1.5$ is evidence of a biological reaction. The high Q_{10} found for neuromuscular synaptic delay by Katz and Miledi[33] was taken as strong evidence in favour of a neuro-transmitter rather than electrical conduction across the synapse. In our experiments the low Q_{10} found for C_{10} suggests that the kinetics of the block it induces is controlled by a purely physical process. This is in keeping with our proposal of a presynaptic site of action (see Chapter 14), and with our observations on C_{10} block in the isolated arm experiments and the effect of blood flow demonstrated by Churchill Davidson and Richardson.[34] The Q_{10} for vecuronium is too high for the onset and offset rate of this block to be controlled by physical events alone. It could result from a binding and unbinding receptor mechanism or from a complex

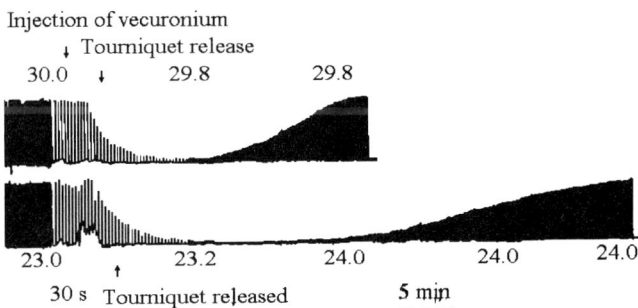

Fig. 15.7 Effect of cold on the onset and offset of vecuronium block in the isolated forearm compared with normothermic control. Note the considerable slowing of onset and recovery by cooling.

Injection of Decamethonium
↓
Tourniquet down
31.0   ↓ 31.0   30.8

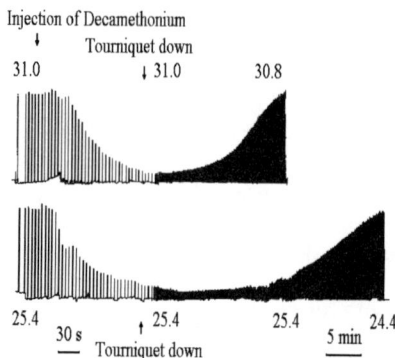

25.4   ↑ 25.4   25.4   24.4
    30 s   5 min
    — Tourniquet down

Fig. 15.8 Effect of cold on the onset and offset of C_{10} block in the isolated forearm. Note the minimal effect of cold on the rate of onset and recovery.

In the upper trace the skin temperature during recovery is 30.8°C, in the lower trace the temperature is between 25.0 and 24.4°C.

The recovery index in the cold arm is 7.5 min and in the warm arm 5.5 min.

The Q_{10} of this experiment is 1.5.

series of physical and chemical events involving a change in entropy. It is unlikely that the Q_{10} would be so high if it were due to buffered diffusion.[35]

This interpretation of our findings fits our observations in the isolated arm following the effect of alterations in blood flow and is strong evidence in favour of biophase binding. When the same experiment was repeated using rocuronium, we found that the Q_{10} of onset was lower than that of vecuronium and nearer that of C_{10} than vecuronium, although the Q_{10} of offset was similar to that of vecuronium. This supports the hypothesis that the onset kinetics of rocuronium block is dependent upon its action at a presynaptic site where biophase binding does not appear to occur, whereas recovery from its block is a function of a postsynaptic effect.

References

1. Holmes PEB, Jenden DJ & Taylor DB. The analysis of the action of curare on neuromuscular transmission. The effect of temperature changes. *J Pharmacol Exp Ther* 1951; **103**: 382–402
2. Cannard TH & Zaimis E. The effect of temperature on the action of neuromuscular blocking drugs in man. *J Physiol (Lond)* 1959; **141**: 112–119
3. Zaimis E, Canard TH & Price HL. Effects of lowered muscle temperature upon neuromuscular blockade in man. *Science* 1958; **128**: 34–35
4. Paton WDM. Possible causes of prolonged apnoea. *Anaesthesia* 1958; **13**: 253
5. Buzello W, Schluerman D, Polmacher T & Spillner G. Unequal effects of cardiopulmonary bypass induced hypothermia on neuromuscular blockade from constant infusion of alcuronium, d-tubocurarine, pancuronium and vecuronium. *Anesthesiology* 1987; **66**: 842–846
6. Feldman SA. (1979) *Muscle Relaxants*, 2nd edn (1979). Philadelphia: WB Saunders, pp. 141–146
7. Thornton RJ, Feldman SA & Blackeney C. (1975) The effect of hypothermia on neuromuscular conduction. In: *Abstracts 5th World Congress Anaesthesiologists*. Amsterdam: Excerpta Medica, p. 12

8. Foldes FF, Kuzo S, Vizi ES & Deery A. The influence of temperature on neuromuscular performance. *J Neural Trans* 1978; **43**: 27–45

9. Miller RD, Van Nyhuis LS & Eger EI II. The effect of temperature on a *d*-tubocurarine blockade and its antagonism by neostigmine. *J Pharmacol Exp Ther* 1975; **195**: 237–244

10. Ham J, Miller RD, Bennet LZ, Matteo RS & Roderick LL. Pharmacokinetics and pharmacodynamics of *d*-tubocurarine during hypothermia in the cat. *Anesthesiology* 1978; **49**: 324

11. England AJ. (1995) Effect of hypothermia on neuromuscular conduction in the rat and guinea pig phrenic nerve diaphragm preparation. MD Thesis, University of London

12. Lucas K. The temperature coefficient of the rate of conduction in nerve. *J Physiol (Lond)* 1908; **37**: 112–121

13. Kostial K & Vouk VB. The influence of temperature on acetylcholine output from sympathetic ganglia. *J Physiol (Lond)* 1956; **132**: 239–241

14. Hubbard JI, Jones SF & Landau EM. The effect of temperature change upon transmitter release, facilitation and post tetanic potentiation. *J Physiol (Lond)* 1971; **216**: 591–609

15. Katz B & Miledi R. The effect of temperature on synaptic delay at the neuromuscular junction. *J Physiol (Lond)* 1965; **118**: 656–670

16. Brust M, Toback S & Benton JG. Some effects of ultrasound and of temperature on contractions of mammalian skeletal muscle. *Arch Physiol Med Rehab* 1969; **50**: 677–694

17. Close R & Hoh JFY. Influence of temperature on isometric contractions of rat skeletal muscle. *Nature* 1968; **217**: 1179–1180

18. Li CL. Effect of cooling on neuromuscular transmission in the rat. *Am J Physiol* 1958; **194**: 200–206

19. Hodgkin AL & Katz B. The effect of temperature on the electrical activity of the giant axon of the squid. *J Physiol (Lond)* 1949; **109**: 240–248

20. Heier T, Caldwell JE, Sharma ML, Grueke LD & Miller RD. Mild intraoperative hypothermia does not change the pharmacodynamics (concentration effect relationship) of vecuronium in humans. *Anesth Analg* 1994; **78**: 973–977

21. d'Hollander AA, Duvaldestin P, Henzel D, Nevelsteen M & Bamblett JP. Variations in pancuronium requirement, plasma concentration and urinary excretion induced by cardiopulmonary bypass with hypothermia. *Anesthesiology* 1983; **58**: 505–509

22. Ham J, Stanski DR, Newfield P & Miller RD. Pharmacokinetics and dynamics of *d*-tubocurarine during hypothermia in humans. *Anesthesiology* 1981; **55**: 631–635

23. Mepham TB & Smith MW. The regulation of amino compound transport across the intestine of goldfish acclimatised to different environment temperatures. *J Physiol (London)* 1966; **186**: 619–626

24. Milton AR. The effect of temperature upon fish cholinesterase. *J Physiol (Lond)* 1958; **142**: 25–26

25. West TC, Frederickson EL & Amory DW. Single fibre recording of the ventricular response to induced hypothermia in anaesthetised dogs. *Circ Res* 1959; **7**: 880

26. Walker SM. The relation of stretch and temperature to contraction of skeletal muscle. *Am J Phys Med* 1960; **39**: 234–238

27. Kelley E & Fry WJ. Isometric twitch tension of frog skeletal muscle as a function of temperature. *Science* 1958; **128**: 200–202

28. Engback J, Skovgaard LT, Friis B, Kahn T & Viby Mogenson J. Monitoring neuromuscular transmission by electromyography stability and temperature dependence of evoked EMG response compared to mechanical twitch recordings in the cat. *Acta Anesthesiol Scan* 1992; **36**: 495–504

29. England AJ, Feldman SA, Redai I, Wu X & Richards K. The effect of moderate hypothermia on recovery of vecuronium neuromuscular block. *Anaesthesia* 1996; (in press)

30. Glavinovic MI, Lawmin JC, Kapural L, Donati F & Bevan DR. Speed of action of various muscle relaxants at the neuromuscular junction binding v buffered diffusion. *J Pharmacol Exp Ther* 1993; **265**: 1181–1186

31. South FE. Phrenic nerve diaphragm preparations in relation to temperature and hibernation. *Am J Physiol* 1961; **200:** 565–571

32. Hill AV. The mode of action of nicotine and curari, determined by the form of the contraction curve and the method of temperature coefficients. *J Physiol (Lond)* 1909; **39:** 361–373

33. Katz B & Miledi R. The measurement of synaptic delay and the time course of acetylcholine release at the neuromuscular junction. *Proc R Soc* 1965; **161:** 483–495

34. Churchill Davidson HC & Richardson AT. Decamethonium iodide (C_{10}). Some observations using electromyography. *Proc R Soc Med* 1952; **45:** 179–183

35. Armstrong DL & Lester HA. The kinetics of tubocurarine action and restricted diffusion. *J Physiol* 1979; **294:** 365

16

Monitoring neuromuscular conduction

The principle involved in monitoring neuromuscular conduction consists of stimulating a major motor nerve and recording the effect it produces in the muscle supplied. This is termed indirect stimulation, as opposed to direct muscle stimulation. For true measurements of the effect of a drug, or change in the physical environment upon neuromuscular conduction, it is necessary to demonstrate that the muscle remains unaffected by the change or the drug. Direct muscle stimulation involves stimulating the muscle itself. Any differences in the response to direct and indirect stimulation represent changes in neuromuscular conduction (see Figs 15.3 and 15.4, Chapter 15). Ideally, direct stimulation should be carried out on curarized muscle to prevent surface conduction of the impulse to the motor end-plate causing a modified indirect response. These strict conditions are difficult to meet except in artificial experimental conditions and it is not unreasonable to assume that drugs that have been demonstrated in animal muscle preparations not to affect muscle contraction will be unlikely to do so in patients. It is therefore usual only to measure the effect of indirect stimulation in human volunteers and patients. Nevertheless, errors can occur if it is not appreciated that changes in muscle contractility may be taking place and these may alter the validity of measurements based on the force of contraction alone.

Change in muscle contractility

The tension developed in a muscle will be affected by its initial degree of stretch. Skeletal muscle, like cardiac muscle, obeys Starling law, with increasing tension being produced during contraction as the muscle is stretched, until uncoupling of the actin–myosin filaments produces contraction failure. It is necessary therefore to make comparative observations under similar degrees of tension. There is no correct tension to use but if tension is to be measured then a load is selected that effectively restricts shortening of the muscle. It is usual to preload the transducer monitoring force by 200 g in man and 20 g in small animal preparations (such as rat diaphragm).

The effect of the rate of stimulus upon the force developed in muscle is apparent at tetanic rates of stimulus, but minor differences occur between

0.1 and 0.5 Hz. These changes are of no significance provided that the preparation is allowed to stabilize at the rate of stimulation selected. Much has been written about the 'correct' rate of stimulation. However, since all single twitch stimuli, whether at 0.1 or 0.5 Hz, are unphysiological, in the sense that they usually do not occur naturally in humans, the rate is obviously of little importance provided stable conditions are established before measurements are made. However, stimulation rates greater than 0.5 Hz increasingly involve presynaptic mechanisms.

In our experience stabilization requires 8–10 min at 0.2 Hz. Since we are usually interested in measuring changes during a period of time it is essential that the same conditions be maintained over that time period and that one demonstrates a return to ±10% of pre-experimental conditions at the conclusion of the test. Degrees of change should always be measured against the initial twitch height and not that obtained upon recovery. It has been suggested that the duration of the stabilization period may markedly affect onset and recovery times using train-of-four (TOF) stimulation.[1] Using strain gauges in both hands of patients and stabilizing one for 5 min and the other for 20 min, we have found identical onset and recovery times in both hands using 0.2 Hz stimulation.[2] We therefore recommend that the twitch response should be used in comparative measurements rather than the TOF, although a recent study using TOF stimulation using the accelograph also failed to demonstrate any effect associated with a 20-min stabilization period.[3]

Post-tetanic enhancement of contractility occurs in directly stimulated muscle and is a separate event from post-tetanic facilitation and post-tetanic 'decurarization' found in partially curarized patients. This small muscle effect can be demonstrated in the absence of any neuromuscular blocking drug and can be difficult to separate from residual block after reversal with an anticholinesterase.

The effect of cooling on muscle contractility is usually to increase muscle contractility, probably by delaying channel closure and encouraging Ca^{2+} flux into the muscle. This effect is opposite to the depressant effect of cooling on neuromuscular conduction and may reduce the net effect observed when a patient's muscle temperature falls. A 10–12% decrease in twitch response is usually observed over a 5°C decrease in temperature (see Chapter 15). This effect is of greater significance if the compound EMG rather than mechanomyography is used.

If one is to avoid confusion in interpreting results and to obtain recovery of twitch force to ±10% of control, it is advisable to keep the muscle within 1°C of its control value. However, we have not found it necessary to use active measures to prevent cooling in muscles that are being stimulated at 0.2 Hz unless the environmental temperature was exceptionally low.

Stimulation conditions for nerve

In most of our experiments we use a 0.2 ms current duration. This is selected as it allows adequate voltage to be administered without the sensation of burning. Larger pulse widths – up to 0.5 ms – risk tissue damage and beyond this duration the stimulus may occur at both the 'make' and 'break' of a square wave current. Shorter pulse widths are used in patient treatments and have the advantages of not stimulating fine nerve fibres such as those carrying the sensation of pain, but they do not always ensure that all motor fibres are stimulated. Using 0.2 ms pulse width with silver–silver chloride skin electrodes placed over cleaned (but not scarified) skin, a voltage of between 90 and 140 V may be required to obtain a supramaximal stimulation. Lower voltages suffice if needle (electroencephalogram) electrodes are used. If needles are used they should be placed just under the skin and parallel to the motor nerve. If they are pointed at the nerve a high charge density at their tip may burn the nerve. Needle electrodes have advantages in that they do not 'dry out' or come unstuck during long experiments and their relationship to the nerve is more consistent than surface electrodes, which can move as the skin slides over the muscle. This is especially likely to occur if the ulnar nerve is stimulated at the elbow.

Whatever method of stimulation is preferred, it is essential that it should be demonstrated to be supramaximal. As the force of contraction will be determined by the number of muscle fibres contracting and this will be 'all or none' for each fibre, it is necessary to be certain at all times that all muscle fibres capable of responding do so. Probably more problems arise due to the use of submaximal nerve stimulation than any other shortcoming. It is sensible to check that the stimulus remains supramaximal during the course of a prolonged procedure.

Rate of stimulation

Recent work in our department has demonstrated the importance of standardizing the rate of stimulation, especially when studying onset times of blocking drugs. We reported that increasing the rate of stimulation from 0.1 to 1.0 Hz reduced the onset time of rocuronium neuromuscular block from 90 to 48 s.[4] Further studies have demonstrated a similar but less marked effect with vecuronium (Fig. 16.1). Although onset time is reduced at higher stimulation frequencies, it has little effect on recovery rate. We have performed studies comparing the effect of increasing frequency of stimulation on 200 stimuli at 0.1, 1 or 2 Hz on the onset of twitch depression by hexamethonium (principally a presynaptic effect), α-bungarotoxin (principally a postsynaptic effect), vecuronium and rocuronium on the rat phrenic nerve diaphragm preparation. The effect was most marked with rocuronium and hexamethonium, less marked with vecuronium and no effect was recorded with α-bungarotoxin (Fig. 16.2). These results support the view that increasing the rate of stimulation, even over this limited range, without increasing the number of stimuli produced a rundown of acetylcholine (ACh) which is in proportion to the action of the drug used at the presynaptic receptors. It suggests that rocuronium has a potent, early blocking action at the presynaptic receptor which is similar to that of a dose of hexamethonium. The doses of all drugs used were sufficient to produce a protest 10% twitch depression in the rat diaphragm. It appears that by comparing the response to 0.1 and 1 Hz

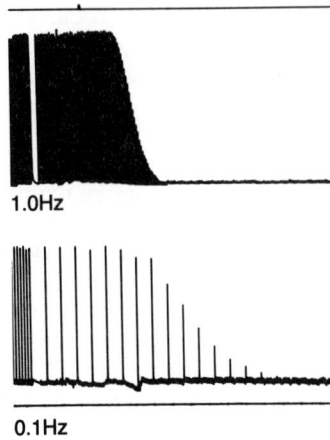

Fig. 16.1 The effect of stimulation frequency on the rate of onset of vecuronium block.

stimulation rate in terms of rate of onset or degree of block developed by a subparalytic dose of drug, it may be possible to assess relative presynaptic actions of different agents.

Methods of recording muscle response

In the laboratory it is possible to monitor single-fibre depolarization and to record it as a single-fibre event using an electromyogram (EMG; Fig. 16.3).

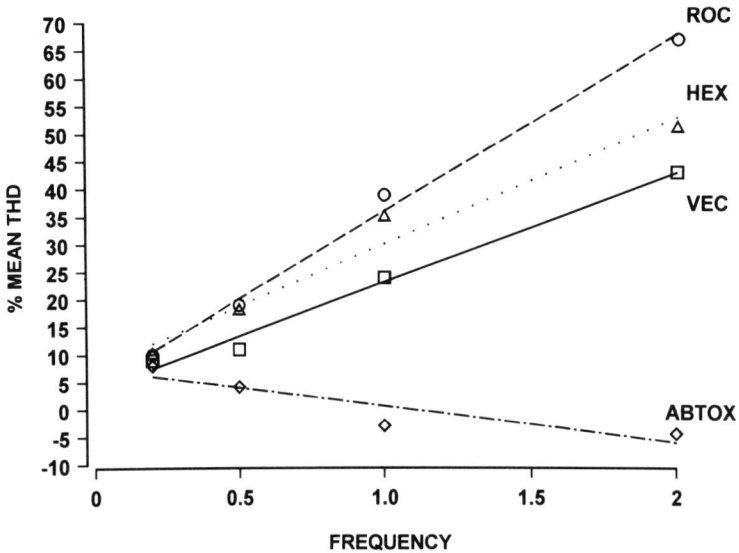

Fig. 16.2 Decrease in twitch tension in rat diaphragm exposed to 10% blocking dose of rocuronium (ROC), hexamethonium (HEX), vecuronium (VEC) and α-bungarotoxin (ABTOX). Effect of rate of stimulation upon 200 stimulations of the phrenic nerve. THD = depression twitch response. (Work in progress Richards K., England A.J., Feldman S.A., Redai I.)

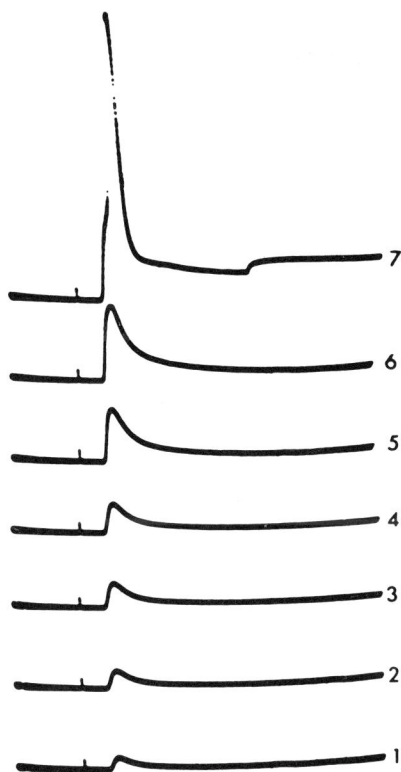

Fig. 16.3 Single-fibre electromyogram during curarization. A series of intracellular end-plate potentials recorded during washout of tubocurare from the end-plate of a frog. The amplitude of the end-plate potential in the lowest trace amounts to only a few millivolts. During the washout end-plate potentials gradually gain in amplitude. In the uppermost trace the critical membrane potential is reached and an action potential is propagated. From Nastuk.[20]

In whole animals and patients it is usual to measure either the tension developed as the muscle contracts or the total electromotive force generated as many fibres become depolarized in response to nerve stimulation – the compound EMG. Both methods have limitations and advantages. In most circumstances they give results of a similar order and similar trends. They are equally easy to interpret. However, it should be appreciated that they measure different modalities associated with neuromuscular conduction.

The mechanomyograph and the electromyogram

Various devices can be used to follow the force produced by muscle contraction subsequent to indirect stimulation. The simplest have utilized water-filled bags taped to the hand and attached to a monometer or tonometer. Some of the early clinical trials with relaxants used the cuff of a sphygmomanometer, half inflated, strapped on to the hand to measure voluntary hand grip weakness.[5] We have used a 20 ml syringe held in the hand with the plunger attached to the thumb to give an indication of neuromuscular block and the return of function. However, for physiological measurement a modified strain gauge system is preferred. The earliest device used by Zaimis *et al.*[6] in her studies in humans adapted a leg calliper. Two strain gauges were used to measure the force developed in dorsiflexion of the foot subsequent to stimulation of the lateral popliteal nerve as it is passed over the head of the fibula. Unfortunately, stimulation in the region of the fibula often causes direct muscle stimulation as well as an indirect response. Devices using the force of contraction of the adductor pollicis muscles have been widely used to follow the response to ulnar nerve stimulation at the wrist. This method of monitoring neuromuscular block was originally suggested by Katz.[7] We prefer a pusher apparatus using either a Statham UC3 force transducer[8] or the rather more robust RS2 bonded strain gauge (originally designed for electronic weighing machines).[9] This type of apparatus is stable, easily balanced and gives a linear response. It does not require the use of an arm board (Fig. 16.4). A 2 kg limit is adequate for twitch or TOF studies, but the force of tetanic stimulation requires use of the 20 kg device. Pulling apparatus with a ring around the thumb such as the Biometer myograph are more difficult to use, have a limited response range and necessitates fixing the arm on a bulky arm board which is too readily disturbed by the surgical team. Contrary to reports, these pieces of equipment are not affected by temperature.[10]

As this apparatus measures force it reflects the number of muscle fibres contracting. A diminution in twitch response following supramaximal nerve stimulation therefore implies that some motor units are not responding whilst others are active. This is caused by insufficient depolarization of the end-plate to trigger an action potential in the more sensitive fibres in the presence of a blocking drug. As the block progresses, more and more neuromuscular junctions will fail to transmit the nerve stimulation and the force of contraction will be reduced.

The compound EMG apparatus, of which the Datex Relaxograph is a good example, measures the electrical activity generated between the two recording electrodes in the muscle studied. Some electrical activity may occur even in those fibres which do not contract and it is the compounding of all electrical activity that produces some of the differences between EMG and mechanical recordings. Both measurements are valid indicators of neuromuscular block.

Twitch, tetanus and train-of-four

Truly physiological studies of neuromuscular block would follow the effect of 30–50 Hz bursts of tetanic stimulus administered for 5 s duration. However, unless a rest period of 5–10 min is used, the effects of post-tetanic potentiation and post-tetanic facilitation of contraction are difficult to separate from the effects of blocking drugs. Tetanic stimulation by direct as opposed to magnetic stimulation of the nerve is very painful and is therefore unsuitable for conscious volunteers. In practice it is easier to

(a)

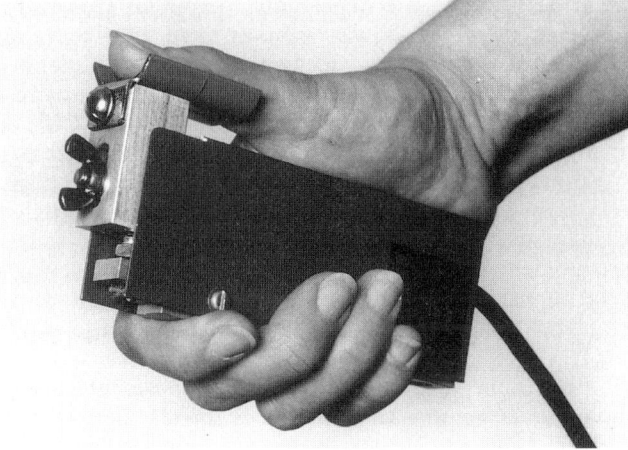

(b)

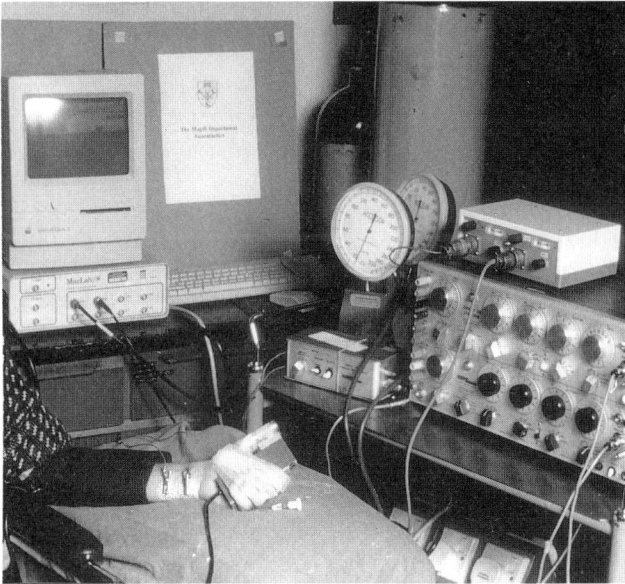

Fig. 16.4 (a) The RS2 strain gauge fitted with thumb cradle for recording the response of the adductor pollicis to ulnar nerve stimulation at the wrist. The thumb is abducted to near 90°. (b) The strain gauge in use. The arm does not need to be fixed to an arm board.

study the effect of single supramaximal twitch stimulation at 0.1 or 0.2 Hz. Whatever rate of stimulation is preferred, it must be used consistently if comparative studies are to be made. Generally a very rapid twitch frequency shortens onset and results in a slightly quicker recovery from neuromuscular block. Thus, repeat 30 Hz stimulation every minute causes more rapid recovery than 0.5 Hz (see Chapter 10). Originally it was suggested that this represented the reversal effect of the increased quantal

ACh to which the receptor was repeatedly[11] exposed. However, in more recent experiments in which it was demonstrated that repeated tetanic stimulation produced a more rapid recovery in the TOF fade, it has been proposed that more rapid rates of stimulation produce a positive feedback on the motor nerve, causing a greater quantal release of ACh[12] (Fig. 4.4). It is evident that using tetanic stimulation produces a greater presynaptic effect than using twitch stimulation and will therefore produce a more rapid recovery from presynaptic block than that seen using single twitches. It has been suggested that, rather than comparing tetanic fade over 5 s, a better measurement to compare the degree of neuromuscular dysfunction would be to measure tetanic tension in 5 s; this can be arrived at by measuring the total area under the tetanic response during a 5 s stimulation.[13]

The TOF stimulation at 2 Hz is some way intermediate between these events. Although it is by no means certain that TOF fade represents presynaptic receptor block as clearly as tetanic fade (50 Hz for 5 s), it is probable that it is mainly influenced by presynaptic events. As a monitor of neuromuscular block it is likely that TOF fade will be more affected by drugs and physical changes that involve major presynaptic events, whereas postsynaptic events will cause more T_1 or single twitch response depression.

Train-of-four

The train-of-four test for residual curarization was introduced by Ali *et al.*[14] and its correlation with residual muscle weakness in humans was demonstrated by Ali and Savarese.[15] The test originated in the observation that patients with myasthenia gravis show a fade of fast twitch response which was maximal between twitch 2 and 8. Because of the parallel between observed tetanic fade and TOF fade,[11] it has been accepted that TOF fade represents a failure of the positive feedback at the presynaptic nicotinic receptors, causing less mobilization of reserve ACh than would be required fully to meet the demands continuing nerve stimulation.

As almost all neuromuscular blocking agents and drugs acting at ACh receptors in the synaptic cleft are capable of acting both at pre- and postsynaptic nicotinic receptor sites (even C_6, regarded as a 'pure' presynaptic blocking drug, will affect postsynaptic receptors in very high doses and α-bungarotoxin is a high-affinity postsynaptic blocking drug which will affect ACh release in high doses), measuring the TOF fade by comparing the ratio of T_4 twitch height to T_1 is a convenient way of testing for residual neuromuscular block. However, there are difficulties in accepting TOF fade itself as it is largely influenced by presynaptic events (see Chapter 10).

It is generally accepted that a TOF fade of less than 30%, i.e. $T_4 > 70\%$ T_1, represents a satisfactory reversal of neuromuscular block.[16] This has been found to correlate well with the patient's ability to maintain a head lift and with ability to cough. Although this has been demonstrated to be a good indication of recovery in practice, it is difficult to reconcile this arbitrary figure with the varying effects of different drugs in their ability to affect ACh release. Wessler *et al.*[17] found that tubocurare produces depression of ACh release to a greater extent than other drugs, whilst atracurium, vecuronium and pancuronium reduce its release by only 20–30%. There are also differences in the rate of onset and offset of TOF fade relative to T_1 during onset of block and during recovery.[18] It rapidly recovers after mivacurium block but does so more slowly following vecuronium and even more slowly after tubocurare.

It is essential therefore to be cautious in interpreting TOF fade in a mechanistic sense, although it remains a useful empirical test for residual curarization.

Double-burst stimulation

Double-burst stimulation has been extensively studied by Engbeck *et al.*[19] It is based upon the more certain pharmacology of post-tetanic facilitation. Post-tetanic facilitation is observed during recovery from all non-depolarizing blocking drugs. It represents the overshoot of ACh production following the positive feedback occurring during tetanic stimulation. As a result, a second stimulus during the period of excess ACh production will cause an enhanced ACh output and a marked response. This makes the difference between the two bursts much easier to recognize than if a single twitch had been used. The advantage of this technique of monitoring recovery from neuromuscular block is that it provides evidence of returning neuromuscular transmission and it is easier to recognize, in the absence of a recorder, than TOF fade during the early recovery of neuromuscular activity. Modifications of this technique, such as the post-tetanic twitch count, utilize the same principles and can provide quantifiable evidence of a progressive recovery from neuromuscular block.

In general, the use of double-burst stimulation or post-tetanic enhancement gives early warning of recovery from neuromuscular block. As such it is particularly useful in monitoring continuous infusion techniques or repeat doses. The TOF fade is a good empirical method of deciding whether there has been sufficient recovery from the block at the end of an operation to allow the patient to be returned to the recovery area.

References

1. McCoy EP, Connolly F, Loan PB & Mirahkur RK. Influence of duration of stimulation on measurement of the onset of neuromuscular block. *Br J Anaesth* 1994; **73:** 264P
2. Redai I, England AJ & Feldman SA. The time taken for stabilization of the muscle twitch does not necessarily affect onset and offset of atracurium. *Br J Anaesth* 1995; **74:** 474P
3. Girling KJ & Mahay RP. (1995) Personal communication
4. Feldman SA & Khaw K. The effect of variations in dose on the action of rocuronium with observations on the effect of the rate of stimulation. *J Anaesthiol* 1995; (in press)
5. Organe GSW, Paton WDM & Zaimis EJ. Preliminary trials of bistrimethylammonium decane and pentene diodide in man. *Lancet* 1949; **1:** 21–25
6. Zaimis E, Cannard TH & Price HL. Effects of lowered body temperature upon neuromuscular block in man. *Science* 1958; **128:** 34–36

7. Katz RL. Comparison of electrical and mechanical recording of spontaneous and evoked muscle activity. *Anesthesiology* 1965; **26:** 204–207

8. Tyrrell MF. The measurement of force of thumb adduction. *Anaesthesia* 1969; **24:** 626–629

9. Campkin NTA, Hood JR & Feldman SA. A modified bonded strain gauge for adductor pollicis mechanomyography. *Anaesthesia* 1993; **48:** 83

10. England AJ, Wu X & Feldman SA. Effect of temperature on the sensitivity of transducers used in human volunteers during neuromuscular stimulation. *Anaesthesia* 1994; **49:** 554

11. Feldman SA & Tyrrell MF. A new theory of the termination of action of the muscle relaxants. 1970; **63:** 692–695

12. Golpinath S, Hood JR, Ulhaq M, Campkin NTA & Feldman SA. Effect of voluntary tetanus on recovery of vecuronium block in isolated forearm. *Anaesthesia* 1993; **48:** 870–872

13. Campkin NTA, Hood JR & Feldman SA. Train of four and 50 Hz tetanus during recovery from neuromuscular block. *Anesth Analg* 1993; **76:** S33

14. Ali HH, Utting JE & Gray C. Stimulus frequency in the detection of neuromuscular blocks in humans. *Br J Anaesth* 1970; **42:** 967–977

15. Ali HH & Savarese JJ. Monitoring neuromuscular function. *Anesthesiology* 1976; **45:** 216–249

16. Viby Mogensen J. Clinical assessment of neuromuscular transmission. *Br J Anaesth* 1982; **54:** 209–223

17. Wessler I, Jung E, Wangenmann K, Vogt T *et al.* Effects of neuromuscular blocking agents on neuronal nicotinic receptors of motor nerves: blockade of nicotinic auto-facilitation and back firing. *Adv Biosci* 1991; **82:** 35–36

18. Harper NJ. (1994) Neuromuscular blockade, measurement and monitoring. In: *Applied Neuromuscular Pharmacology*, Pollard BJ (ed.). Oxford: Oxford University Press, p. 326

19. Engbeck J, Ostergaard D & Viby Mogensen J. Double burst stimulation (DBS). A new pattern of nerve stimulation to identify residual curarization. *Br J Anaesth* 1989; **62:** 274–278

20. Nastuk WL. The electrical activity of the muscle cell membrane at the neuromuscular junction. *J Cell Comp Physiol* 1953; **42:** 249–256

17

The ideal muscle relaxant

There is general agreement about the properties required by an ideal muscle relaxant drug. Having proposed an explanation of neuromuscular block and how it is reversed, it is possible to postulate how the conditions required by the ideal drug might be achieved.

Site of action

Ideally, muscle relaxation would be achieved by depressing the most sensitive part of the transmission process between the nerve and the muscle; this implies blocking neuromuscular conduction. This could, in theory, be achieved by interfering with acetylcholine (ACh) formation, its storage, mobilization and release or by antagonizing ACh action at pre- and postsynaptic ACh receptor sites. Efforts to depress ACh formation by agents such as hemicholinium or vesamicol produce a rundown of neuromuscular transmission which is too slow to be of practical use in anaesthesia.[1] Drugs which interfere with ACh storage and mobilization, such as botulinus toxin, are too long-acting to be practical for clinical anaesthesia.[2] However, both these mechanisms may find a place in the control of the long-term painful muscle spasm associated with degenerative nervous disease. At the moment only botulinus toxin is used for this purpose. Drugs which act principally presynaptically, such as pentamethonium, unfortunately all possess ganglion-blocking properties in lower doses than that required to produce neuromuscular block, which makes them unsuitable for use as muscle relaxants. Drugs acting solely at the postsynaptic sites, such as α-bungarotoxin, are necessarily slow in onset and offset.

It is therefore likely that future developments will continue to concentrate on producing drugs that act at both the pre- and postsynaptic sites in order to produce the ideal muscle relaxant. The synergism resulting from this dual action should, in theory, increase the rate of onset of block and reduce the dose of drug required to produce muscle relaxation. It is probable that all neuromuscular blocking drugs act at both pre- and postsynaptic sites to a varying extent,[3] but whilst we have considerable evidence of their postsynaptic action we lack similar information regarding the rate and effectiveness of their presynaptic activity.

The ideal drug

The ideal muscle relaxant would have the following properties:

Onset

Full neuromuscular block should be produced in 40–60 s, i.e. two to three times the circulation time. This begs the question as to whether it is more important to paralyse the muscle of the larynx before those of the adductor pollicis or masseter. In practice, if the adductor pollicis muscle is 80–90% paralysed, intubation of the trachea will not be impaired even if there is some movement of the vocal cords. If it takes 90 s to achieve paralysis to a 0.1 Hz stimulation of the adductor pollicis there will be at least a 10% failure rate of intubation at 40–60 s and a further 10% of patients with less than excellent conditions for intubation. This is less than ideal.

Ease of reversal

The safety of the neuromuscular blocking drugs lies in the ability to reverse their actions completely, either by spontaneous recovery or with the aid of an anticholinesterase drug. It would theoretically be better to have a drug whose action reversed spontaneously and instantly once its administration was stopped as this would avoid any complication resulting from the use of neostigmine (such as its effect on gut anastomosis[4]). However, the morbidity following the correct use of neostigmine is very low and the need for its adminstration might not be significantly reduced, as the effect of drug at the receptor clearly outlasts the decline in its plasma concentration (see Chapter 5).

The possibility of inadequate, incomplete or temporary reversal of the action of a neuromuscular blocking drug must be the most serious disadvantage in normal clinical practice. However, it must be admitted that, even today, techniques are advocated in some centres using drugs in a manner that makes complete reversal difficult. These techniques can only be justified when the patients are to be electively ventilated postoperatively. These techniques, whilst practical in skilled hands, have little scientific justification.

Duration of action

Savarese and Kitz in a much quoted editorial[5] described the need for three types of neuromuscular blocking agents with duration of action lasting from 10 to 60 min. Whilst this approach would fulfil anaesthetists' requirements, it is also possible to achieve adequate flexibility of duration of block using a short-acting drug that can be continuously infused or a long-acting drug whose action could be safely and completely terminated by an anticholinesterase within 5 min of administration. Both these approaches would give similar flexibility. A continuously infused drug is pharmacokinetically and scientifically more appealing; however, a longer-acting drug, such as Org 9487, whose action could be terminated, would be more convenient, less complicated to use and cheaper.

Specificity of action

It would be difficult to market any muscle relaxant that had significant side-effects in doses up to five times the ED_{95}. We have come to accept that neuromuscular blocking drugs will not influence blood pressure and pulse rate nor will they or their metabolites affect the function of the central nervous system, kidneys or liver. It is arguable that we have drugs that are 'too pure' and it has been suggested that some vagolytic action might be an advantage to offset the actions of the potent analgesics and some volatile agents which are generally vagotonic.

Histamine release

Whilst drugs that release histamine are more limited and less flexible than drugs that do not do so, the widespread safe use of tubocurare, atracurium and mivacurium is testament to the relative unimportance of this effect when it is so small that it does not produce hypotension in up to three times the ED_{95} dose. The limitation is evident in the restriction that has to be placed on the size of any bolus compared to that of a drug that does not release histamine. It is not uncommon to administer vecuronium in up to $5 \times ED_{95}$ in order to achieve either a longer action or better intubating condition; this technique could not be used if it released histamine. The development of cisatracurium, a drug which in many aspects is less attractive than the parent atracurium, is justified as it does not release histamine in clinical doses.

It is evident that there is little association between drugs that release histamine and the incidence of anaphylactoid reactions. Atracurium has a low incidence of anaphylactoid reactions, whereas suxamethonium, which does not release histamine, has the highest incidence of serious reactions of this nature.

Onset of action

Various methods have been suggested for increasing the rate of onset of non-depolarizing drugs, including decreasing the potency and increasing dosage. These are described in Chapter 9. There must be a limit to the usefulness of both these approaches. Decreasing drug potency in order to reduce the onset time, by producing a more rapid dissociation of the drug from binding sites, has its limit as the dissociation will become so rapid that it is no longer bound and is a less effective competitor for ACh. When this occurs the amount of block produced will parallel the synaptic cleft and plasma drug concentration. Following bolus administration the drug concentration in the plasma may rise sufficiently to produce a block but, unless this is maintained it will decline, as redistribution of drug occurs, resulting in a rapid waning of the blocking effect. Only a continuous infusion of the drug at a rate that will maintain a plasma to synapse concentration equilibrium sufficiently high to compete with ACh will maintain a block. This predictable consequence of very low potency has been demonstrated in practice with the aminosteroid Org 7617.[6] The low potency necessitates using vast amounts of drug to maintain an effective synaptic cleft concentration of the agent. This in turn increases the risk of side-effects, from both the parent compound and from its metabolites. It may also produce delayed plasma clearance of drug. It is evident that it cannot be the potency itself that is responsible for rapid onset, nor is it a question of a higher plasma to synaptic cleft concentration gradient resulting from the high doses used, because the concentration of a weak drug required in the synaptic cleft in order to produce a given effect is necessarily much greater than with a more potent one which competes more effectively with ACh at the receptor.

A very high concentration gradient between plasma extracellular fluid (ECF) and receptor (or even water bath, in case of the phrenic nerve diaphragm preparation) will produce rapid onset as it will rapidly overwhelm the limits of the binding compartment. Once this is achieved any additional drug will not be bound and will act as though it had a negligible K_D, being more readily available to compete with ACh at the receptor site in a log dose–effect relationship. However, in clinical practice this only occurs with excessive doses of drug. In the case of vecuronium this needs a dose in excess of $10 \times ED_{95}$ dose.

Evidence has been presented that suxamethonium and decamethonium (C_{10}) owe their rapid onset of block to a presynaptic site of action.[7-9] It is tempting to suggest that the more rapid onset of action of rocuronium and AN9040 (an experimental aminosteroid drug)[10] is due to a similar early action at a presynaptic site, coupled with a slower onset of postsynaptic block.[11,12] Evidence to support this proposition comes from the train-of-four (TOF) fade produced by both these drugs within 60 s of an ED_{50} dose[13] (Fig. 17.1) and the rapid onset of action of a $2 \times ED_{90}$ dose of rocuronium (45 s) observed when a 1 Hz stimulation rate is used rather than 0.1 Hz.[14] This additional early site of action of rocuronium would help explain why its onset of action is so rapid when compared to its offset (see Chapter 10). The onset–offset profile of this drug lies outside that of other drugs studied, suggesting a different or extra mode of action. A further indication that rocuronium differs from other non-depolarizing drugs in its onset is the inability to use rocuronium successfully to prime

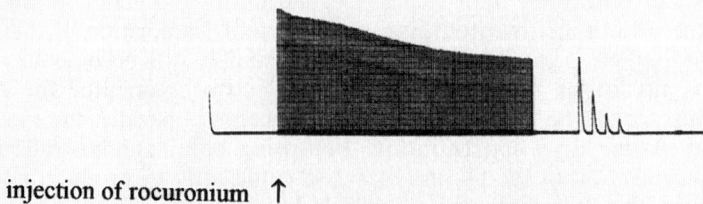

injection of rocuronium ↑

Fig. 17.1 Onset of pronounced train-of-four fade with minimal T_1 block by rocuronium. This suggests a major presynaptic component to rocuronium block.

itself in order to produce the accelerated onset of action seen with all other non-depolarizing drugs.[15] It is tempting to ascribe its inability to prime itself to its already rapid onset rate (90 s in $2 \times ED_{95}$ dose); however, this onset time can be reduced to under 60 s by priming with vecuronium (see Chapter 15). Rocuronium priming will reduce the onset time of vecuronium block, particularly if the dose of rocuronium used produces TOF fade.[16] It is possible that an early rapid presynaptic effect of rocuronium acts to speed the onset of the postsynaptic block by reducing the ACh output and hence the level of occupancy of the ACh receptors required to produce neuromuscular block.

If this theory is correct then it points to the development of non-depolarizing drugs in the future, with a significant presynaptic effect in order to achieve an onset time comparable with suxamethonium.

Ease of reversal

It is evident that a consequence of biophase binding is that the prerequisite for easy complete reversal of non-depolarizing neuromuscular block is a rapid reduction in the plasma concentration of the drug. With a bolus dose of $1 \times ED_{95}$ dose of most non-depolarizing drugs, a rapid reduction in plasma level occurs due to redistribution to non-active sites in the liver, kidney and spleen. For gallamine, suxamethonium and aminosteroid relaxants, rapid redistribution also occurs to cartilage, whereas tubocurare is also distributed in the salivary glands.[17] The rapidity of this redistribution, which produces the initial sharp decline in plasma level observed in pharmacokinetic studies and described as the initial distribution volume, is revealed in autoradiographic studies[17–19] (Fig. 17.2). It is puzzling why these highly positively charged molecules should enter the cells of the liver and kidney with such facility and why they should remain sequestered there for many hours. It is of interest that a high density of drug may appear rapidly in the cartilage of the intervertebral discs and tracheal cartilage in spite of their very poor blood supply.

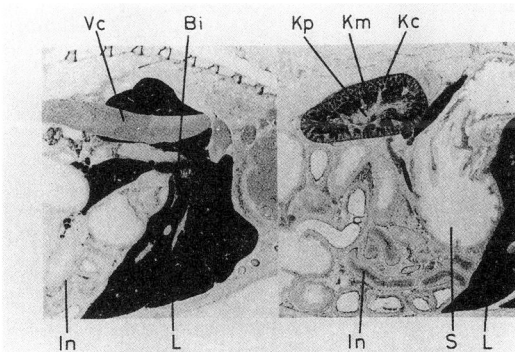

Fig. 17.2 Early redistribution of vecuronium (VC) to liver (L), kidney (K) and bile (Bi) produces a rapid initial decay in plasma concentration. After Waser et al.[38]

It reflects the rapidity with which the drugs pass into the ECF and the avidity of their binding to these non-active sites.

When higher doses of drug ($>ED_{95}$) are administered, metabolism, excretion and secondary redistribution may assist in reducing the plasma level of drug once the redistribution phase is completed (Fig. 17.3). This causes the slower β phase of the plasma concentration curve.

Metabolism

Rapid hydrolysis by cholinesterase causes the lowering of the plasma concentration of suxamethonium and mivacurium in 3–4 min. As this is a log dose effect following first-order kinetics, the higher the dose, the faster the rate of metabolism until the point of enzyme saturation is reached. This form of metabolism will also result in a long plasma concentration 'tail' but this occurs at levels that are too low to be of clinical significance. Enzymatic hydrolysis also occurs *in vitro* with atracurium; however this appears to be at a higher rate in the plasma of some animals (i.e. the rat) than in humans. Figures of the proportion of drug hydrolysed in humans are inconsistent due to the variety of methodologies used, the differing concentrations of the drug, and variations in the relative content of the main isomers in the sample.[20–22] Of the 10 possible isomers of atracurium, the cis–cis isomer, which is to be marketed as cisatracurium, undergoes least hydrolysis.

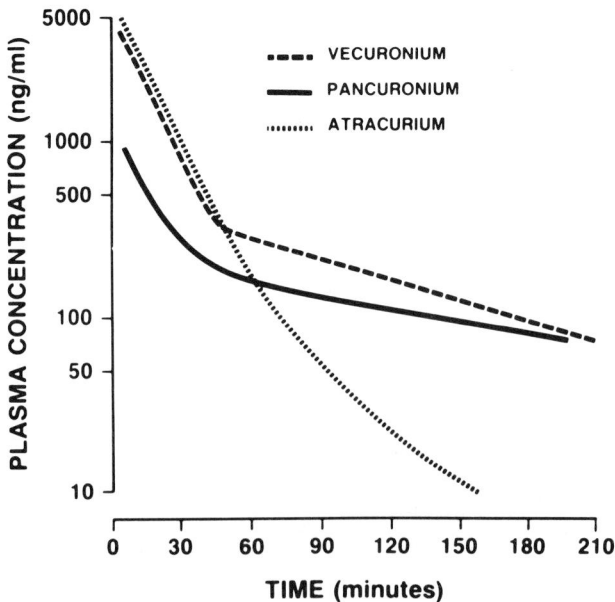

Fig. 17.3 Plasma decay curves of three muscle relaxants. Note the typical biphasic curve for pancuronium and vecuronium, indicating a rapid α phase of redistribution and a slower β phase of metabolism and excretion. Atracurium does not show this effect, as metabolism and Hofmann elimination produce a rapid β phase. From Miller *et al.*[39]

The aminosteroid drugs all undergo deacetylation and oxidation in the liver. The 3 and 17 acetyl groups of vecuronium and pancuronium are metabolized to the hydroxy and acetoxy derivatives[23,25,26] (Fig. 17.4). Rocuronium, which has no acetyl group in the 3 position, is likely to undergo only limited metabolism. The metabolites are then excreted in the bile and the urine. The percentage of drug metabolized in this way may vary from individual to individual and probably depends upon dose of drug, the duration of its administration and the liver blood flow, as well as the level of liver P_{450} isozyme activity. As much as 30% of an injected dose of vecuronium may be metabolized in this fashion.[24-27]

Hofmann degradation

Atracurium is unique in that it undergoes Hofmann degradation.[28] This process occurs in the presence of the reverse ester bond contained in atracurium. It produces electron transport along the methyl chain until it causes rupture of the ammonium bond. It occurs more readily in the presence of an alkaline medium. The metabolism produces a terminal methyl group on one fragment of the molecule and a tertiary ammonium on the other. In this manner the bisquaternary atracurium becomes mono-quarternary and inactive, whilst the moiety split from the parent molecule in the tertiary ammonium form is the compound laudanosine. This is a physical process obeying zero-order kinetics and probably accounts for the greater part of the plasma clearance of atracurium in humans. It is speeded up by alkalization caused by hyperventilation.

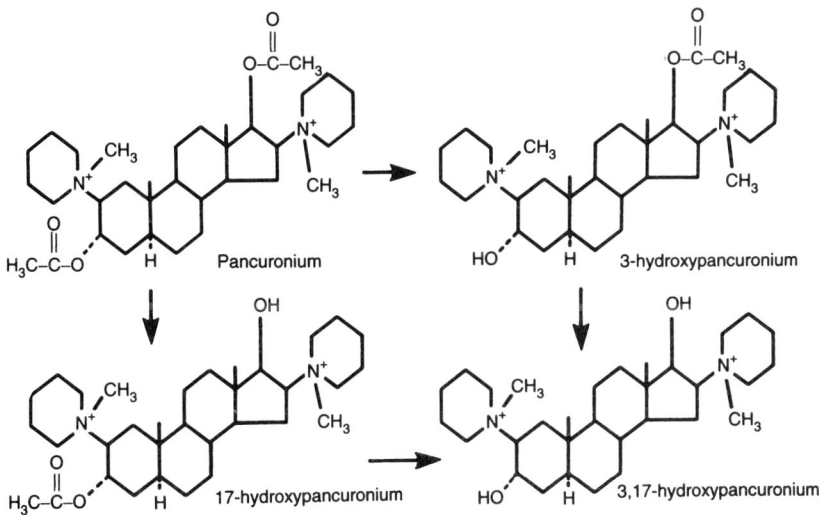

Fig. 17.4 Metabolic pathways for pancuronium. Metabolism at the 3 and 17 groups is similar for vecuronium.

Sequestration

Some drugs have such a rapid hepatic uptake that they are virtually cleared from the plasma following injection into the hepatic artery (Fig. 17.5).[24] On a purely physical basis, one would expect this process to be accelerated by increasing fat solubility; however, rocuronium, which is slightly less fat-soluble than vecuronium, has a greater propensity for sequestration in the liver. It is this property that helps to account for the low recovery rate (less than 30%) of rocuronium and its derivatives 12 h after twice the ED_{95} dose has been administered.

Excretion

Renal excretion

All the neuromuscular blocking drugs are concentrated in the kidney and excreted in the urine. The amount of drug recovered from the urine depends upon the dose of drug administered and the efficacy of other alternative methods of plasma clearance. Drugs such as gallamine[18] and C_{10} appear to depend almost entirely on renal excretion; pancuronium and alcuronium, metacurine and doxacurium[29] do so to a lesser extent, whilst significant alternative pathways exist for clearing tubocurare and vecuronium from the plasma. Drugs such as atracurium, mivacurium and suxamethonium are usually all cleared from the plasma by metabolic pathways in the absence of renal function, although about 10% of atracurium is normally recoverable from the urine.

Biliary excretion

The aminosteroids are all subject to biliary excretion, either as the parent drug or as the metabolite. The amount excreted in this way varies greatly

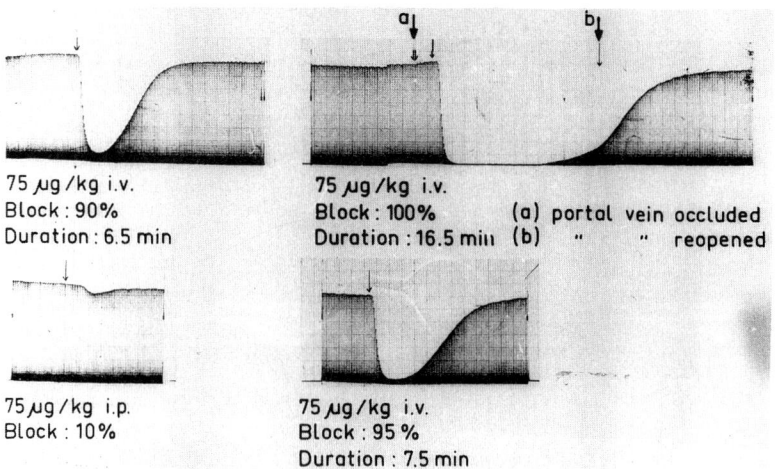

75 μg/kg i.v.
Block : 90%
Duration : 6.5 min

75 μg/kg i.v.
Block : 100%   (a) portal vein occluded
Duration : 16.5 min (b)   "   "   reopened

75 μg/kg i.p.
Block : 10%

75 μg/kg i.v.
Block : 95%
Duration : 7.5 min

Fig. 17.5 Injection of the experimental drug Org 6368 into the portal vein (lower left panel) produces little effect. Injection when the portal vein is occluded and the liver blood flow is reduced produces a prolonged effect (upper right panel).

from one patient to another but this pathway of excretion appears to be of greatest significance following the administration of vecuronium.[30] Rocuronium has been reported to be excreted in the gut, presumably as a result of biliary excretion.

In the absence of renal excretion it has been demonstrated that up to 34% of an injected dose of tubocurare can be recovered from bile in dogs. It is probable that biliary and salivary excretion are minor but significant alternative pathways for the excretion of this drug in normal circumstances.[17]

Significance of various methods of lowering plasma concentration of drug

Each method of plasma clearance has disadvantages and advantages. The disadvantages of metabolism are the occurrence of an active or toxic metabolite and the possibility of the absence of an enzyme system necessary for metabolism.

Metabolism

The 3 hydroxy derivative of vecuronium and pancuronium has been demonstrated to possess about 50% of the neuromuscular blocking potency of its parent compound. The 17 hydroxy and the 3–17 deacetoxy derivatives are very weak blockers and are of little significance. As the half-life of the 3 hydroxy derivative is much longer than that of the parent compound, accumulation of metabolites can occur and this has been suggested as the cause of the difficulty in reversing the action of long-standing vecuronium infusions in patients in the intensive care unit.[31]

Laudanosine, the by-product of the Hofmann degeneration of atracurium, is a central nervous system stimulant allied to ematine. Although no proven case of it accumulating in sufficient quantity in the plasma to cause convulsions has been described, there is evidence from animal experiments that it may reach levels that are analeptic, causing an increase in the minimum alveolar concentration requirements of anaesthetic agents, especially if renal excretion is impaired. However, even in renal failure, levels of laudonosine approaching the 10–15 mmol/l necessary to produce convulsions have not been found.[32]

In the case of suxamethonium and mivacurium, a reduction in the level of plasma cholinesterase will prolong the presence of drug in the blood and result in protracted paralysis.[40,41] Eventually the drug will be excreted in the kidneys but this may take several hours following a $2 \times ED_{95}$ dose of mivacurium.

Sequestration

As the sequestration sites for the drug become filled, the concentration gradient between these acceptor sites and the plasma will be reduced, resulting in a decrease in the rate of plasma clearance of drug. Although this will only occur after large doses or the continuous infusion of the drug, it will result in a reduction in the clearance rate of drug and a marked cumulative effect.

Excretion

Biliary excretion of drug is variable as it depends on liver blood flow and function and hence the rate of clearance by this means is unpredictable.

Renal clearance is subject to being affected by changes in renal blood flow as a result of fluid load, anaesthesia and diseases affecting the kidney.

Specificity of action

The autonomic nervous system blocking effect of curare which, although weak, can produce hypotension and a fall in peripheral resistance, was considered a major disadvantage, especially in the early days of cardiac surgery when maintenance of venous return was required for safe operation upon diseased mitral and aortic valves.

Originally suxamethonium, which produces autonomic excitement in some animals, was passed over in favour of suxaethonium until it was appreciated that it had little autonomic effect in humans. Pancuronium was introduced as the agent of choice for cardiac surgery as it did not produce a fall in peripheral resistance.[33] However, pancuronium produces tachycardia by vagolysis and inhibition of vagal modulation of the sympathetic input to the sinoatrial node. In addition, pancuronium blocks the reuptake of noradrenaline, thus producing a cocaine-like effect, causing vasoconstriction and tachycardia, especially when used during light anaesthesia.[34-36] In order to modify this response it is common practice to use either large doses of opiates or deep anaesthesia to limit the release of catecholamines consequent to endotracheal intubation and surgical stimulation.

The close link between drugs that affect nicotinic and muscarinic receptors is not surprising in view of the common sensitivity to ACh. It was best demonstrated by the early studies of the bisquarternary polymethylene series.[37] In these studies it was demonstrated that extending the number of methyl groups in the chain between the two quaternary amino groups from 6 to 10 changes it from a muscarinic blocker, causing ganglionic blockade and presynaptic block of ACh release, to a depolarizing neuromuscular blocking drug.

Today no drug causing significant autonomic effect would be acceptable in clinical practice.

Histamine release

The benzylisoquinolium compounds all appear to cause histamine release. Provided that this effect does not cause hypotension when the drug is administered in clinical doses (up to $3 \times ED_{95}$). It has not been found to be a great disadvantage. Histamine release has not been demonstrated to be associated with any increase in morbidity or mortality. The cis–cis isomer of atracurium has a much weaker effect on histamine release and it is being developed for clinical use because of this property.

References

1. Marshall IG. Studies on the blocking action of 2 (4-phenylpiperidino)-cyclohexano (AH 5183). *Br J Pharmacol* 1970; **38:** 503–516
2. Marshall IG. The effects of some hemicholinium like substances on the chick biventer cervicis muscle. *Eur J Pharmacol* 1968; **2:** 258–264
3. Foldes FF. (1957) Muscle relaxants. In: *Anesthesiology.* Springfield, Illinois: Charles C Thomas
4. Bell CMA & Lewis CB. Effect of neostigmine on integrity of ileorectal anastomoses. *Br Med J* 1968; **111:** 587–588
5. Savarese JJ & Kitz RJ. Does clinical anaesthesia need new neuromuscular blocking drugs? *Anesthesiology* 1975; **42:** 236–239
6. Wierda JMKH, Proost JH, Muir AW & Marshall RJ. Design of drugs for rapid onset. *Anaesth Pharmacol Rev* 1993; **1:** 57–68
7. Feldman SA, Fauvel NJ & Harrop-Griffiths AW. (1990) The onset of neuromuscular blockade. In: *Neuromuscular Blocking Agents, Past, Present and Future.* Bowman WC, Denissen PAF & Feldman SA (eds). Holland: Excerpta Medica, pp. 44–52
8. Fauvel NJ. Onset of neuromuscular bloc, the effect of biophase delay. *Anaesth Pharm Rev* 1993; **1:** 44–49
9. Feldman SA & Hood JR. Depolarizing neuromuscular block. A presynaptic mechanism? *Acta Anesthesiol Scand* 1994; **38:** 535–541
10. Munday IT & Jones RN. AN9040. Effect of $2 \times ED_{95}$ dose. *Br J Anaesth* 1993; **70:** 480
11. England AJ, Panikkar K, Redai I *et al.* Onset–offset relationships. Is rocuronium an exception? *Br J Anaesth* 1995; **50:** S10–S13
12. Feldman SA & England AJ. (1995) Pharmacology of neuromuscular transmission. In: *Current Opinions in Anesthesiology* Wood M (ed.). London: Rapid Science, pp. 351–356
13. Wierda JMKH, de Wit APM, Kuizenga K & Agoston S. Clinical observations on the neuromuscular blocking action of Org 9426, a new steroidal non-depolarizing agent. *Br J Anaesth* 1990; **64:** 521–523
14. Feldman SA & Khaw K. The effect of dose on the action of rocuronium and on the effect of the rate of stimulation. *Eur J Anaesthesiol* 1995; **12** (suppl 11)
15. Foldes FF. (1990) The clinical pharmacology of Org 9426. In: *Neuromuscular Blocking Agents, Past, Present and Future.* Bowman WC, Denissen PAF & Feldman SA (eds). Holland: Excerpta Medica, pp. 171–182
16. Feldman SA & Redai I. Rocuronium as a priming agent. *Eur J Anaesthesiol* 1995; **12** (suppl 11): 12–15
17. Cohen EN, Hood N & Golling R. Use of whole body autoradiography for determining uptake and distribution of labelled muscle relaxants in the rat. *Anesthesiology* 1968; **21:** 987–991
18. Feldman SA, Cohen EN & Golling R. The excretion of gallamine in the dog. *Anesthesiology* 1969; **30:** 593–597
19. Cohen EN, Carbascio A & Fleischeli G. The distribution and fate of *d*-tubocurarine. *J Pharmacol Exp Ther* 1965; **147:** 120–125
20. Fisher DM, Canfell PC, Fahey MR *et al.* Elimination of atracurium in humans: contribution of Hofmann elimination and ester hydolysis versus organ bound elimination. *Anesthesiology* 1986; **65:** 6–12
21. Ward S, Boheimer N, Weatherley BC *et al.* Pharmacokinetics of atracurium and its metabolites in patients with normal renal function and in patients with renal failure. *Br J Anaesth* 1987; **59:** 697–706
22. Chapple DJ & Clarke JS. Pharmacological action of breakdown products of atracurium and related substances. *Br J Anaesth* 1983; **55:** 11–14
23. Booij LHDJ, Vree TB, Jurkans F *et al.* Pharmacokinetics and pharmacodynamics of the muscle relaxant drug ORG NC45 and each of its metabolites in dogs. *Anaesthetist* 1982; **30:** 329–333

24. Bencinin AF, Scaf AHJ, Agoston S *et al*. Distribution of vecuronium bromide in the cat. *Br J Anaesth* 1985; **57**: 782–789

25. Bencinin AF, Hoawertjes CM & Agoston S. Effects of hepatic uptake of vecuornium and its metabolites on their neuromuscular blocking actions in the cat. *Br J Anaesth* 1985; **57**: 789–795

26. Merrett RA, Thompson CW & Webb FW. *In vitro* degradation of atracurium in human plasma. Br J Anaesth 1983; **55**: 61–66

27. Sohn YJ, Bencini AF, Scaf AHJ *et al*. Comparative pharmacokinetics and dynamics of vecuronium and pancuronium in anaesthetised patients. *Anesth Analg* 1986; **65**: 233–239

28. Stenlake JB, Waigh RD, Urwin J *et al*. Atracurium; conception and inception. *Br J Anaesth* 1983; **55**: 53–60

29. Mellinghoff H, Diefenbach C & Buzello W. (1990) The clinical pharmacology of doxacurium. In: *Neuromuscular Blocking Agents, Past, Present and Future*. Bowman WC, Denissen PAF & Feldman SA (eds). Holland: Excerpta Medica, pp. 79–83

30. Soh YJ, Bencini A, Scaf AHJ *et al*. Pharmacokinetics of vecuronium in man. *Anesthesiology* 1982; **57**: A256

31. Miller RD. (1990) Pharmacokinetics of neuromuscular blocking drugs in intensive care patients. In: *Neuromuscular Blocking Agents, Past, Present and Future*. Bowman WC, Denissen PAF & Feldman SA (eds). Holland: Excerpta Medica, pp. 117–125

32. Lanier WL, Hilde JH & Michenfelder JD. The cerebral effects of pancuronium and atracurium in halothane anesthetised dogs. *Anesthesiology* 1985; **63**: 589–597

33. Baird WLM & Reid AM. The neuromuscular blocking properties of a new steroid compound; pancuronium bromide. *Br J Anaesth* 1967; **39**: 775–780

34. Loh L. The cardiovascular effects of pancuronium bromide. *Anaesthesia* 1970; **25**: 356–363

35. Stoetling RK. The haemodynamic effects of pancuronium and *d*-tubocurarine in anesthetised patients. *Anesthesiology* 1976; **36**: 612–615

36. Barnes PK, Brindle Smith G, White WD *et al*. Comparison of the effects of ORG NC45 and pancuronium bromide on the heart rate and arterial pressure in anaesthetised man. *Br J Anaesth* 1982; **54**: 435–439

37. Paton WDM & Zaimis EJ. The pharmacological actions of the polymethylene bismethyl ammonium salts. *Br J Pharmacol* 1949; **4**: 381

38. Waser PG, Wiederkehr A, Chang Sin-Ren & Kaiser-Schönenberger E. Kinetics and metabolism of ^{14}C-vecuronium in rats and mice. In: *Muscle Relaxants – Therapeutic Margins*. Agoston S, Bergman H, Schwartz S & Steinbereithner K (eds). Vienna: Verlag W. Mandrick

39. Miller RD, Rupp SM & Fisher DM. Clinical pharmacology of vecuronium and atracurium. *Anesthesiology* 1984; **61**: 444–453

18

The muscle relaxant drugs

Of the present available neuromuscular blocking drugs, suxamethonium is the only depolarizing drug in common use. This drug, together with pancuronium, tubocurare, vecuronium, atracurium, mivacurium and rocuronium, will be assessed in this chapter. The properties of all these drugs are well known and only those aspects that command particular attention because of their usefulness, or the specific danger they present, will be considered.

Suxamethonium

Suxamethonium possesses the unique characteristics of rapid onset of action accompanied by the desirable property of a very brief duration of action. This ensures its continued usefulness in spite of it having many disadvantages.

Although classified as a depolarizing drug, there is little doubt that it has a major presynaptic action[1] causing antidromic firing and repetitive after-discharge following motor nerve stimulation and phase II block.[2,3]

More doses of suxamethonium have been administered than any other single muscle relaxant and, although it has been associated with more anaesthetic deaths than any other relaxant per dose used, the incidence of side-effects is still very low. However, because it is more hazardous than any other relaxant, the risk involved in its use must be counterbalanced by a benefit to the patient.

Minor disadvantages

1 *Muscle pains.* Suxamethonium myalgia is especially common after low doses of induction agent and early ambulation.[4] It can be mitigated by prior administration of a small 'taming' dose of non-depolarizing drug.[5]
2 *Fasciculations.* Often, but not necessarily, associated with myalgia,[6] they can be reduced by large doses of induction drugs, a small dose of non-depolarizing agent, by diazepam and by administering a 'taming' dose of 0.1 mg/kg suxamethonium 2 min before the definitive doses.[7] Diazepam and self-taming do not effectively reduce the incidence of myalgia.

3 *Masseteric spasm.* This occurs in fewer than 1% of patients, even in the absence of fasciculations.

4 *Myoglobinuria.*[8] This is usually subclinical but in a few patients, usually exhibiting marked muscle spasm, myoglobinuria is macroscopic and obvious.

5 *Prolonged action.*[9] Because suxamethonium is hydrolysed by plasma cholinesterase, it is usually rapidly cleared from the plasma in spite of the relatively high doses used. Any deficiency in plasma cholinesterase, either congenital or acquired, will result in a prolonged action of the drug. In the absence of normal plasma cholinesterase the duration of block is usually in excess of 2 h and recovery is accompanied by evidence of phase II block.

6 *Raised intraocular pressure.*[10] Although much is made of the risk of the rise in intraocular pressure that accompanies the use of suxamethonium, the effect is usually short-lived (about 5 min) and seldom greater than the effect of a good cough. It can be modified by prior administration of a non-depolarizing drug but this cannot be relied upon in all cases. It is reasonable to avoid its use in patients in whom this transient increase in intraocular pressure presents a serious risk.

7 *Raised intragastric pressure.*[11,12] The risk of regurgitation of stomach contents due to the rise in intragastric pressure is more theoretical than real. Most cases of regurgitation of stomach contents after suxamethonium have been due to attempts to intubate before relaxation has occurred.

8 *Second-dose bradycardia.* It remains a mystery as why suxamethonium should not cause bradycardia with the first dose administered but will do so, especially in adult patients who have not been premedicated with atropine, when a second dose is administered 2–3 min after the first.[13] The bradycardia may be so severe as to cause asystole for up to 2 min. This is a potentially serious complication of repeated use. It is puzzling why the effect of a second dose of suxamethonium should be so much more active at the sinoatrial node in the heart whilst tachyphylaxis produces resistance at the neuromuscular junction.

Major disadvantages

1 *Cardiac arrest.*[14–17] Even in normal circumstances, suxamethonium produces a very small but detectable shift of potassium from inside the cell to the extracellular fluid (ECF). Under certain conditions this effect is massive and the sudden rise in extracellular K^+ may produce cardiac arrest. This is best documented following denervation injury and in paraplegics (Fig. 18.1). As the extent of the K^+ shift is proportional to the number of denervated muscle fibres, it has most frequently been observed following widespread denervation such as that following cord transection. The cause of this effect is believed to be due to the loss of calcitonin gene-related peptide secreted prejunctionally. As a result there is a loss of the focus of acetylcholine receptor (AChR) at the synapse and the widespread presence of perijunctional receptors on the muscle surface. As the half-life of a receptor is about 3 days in humans,

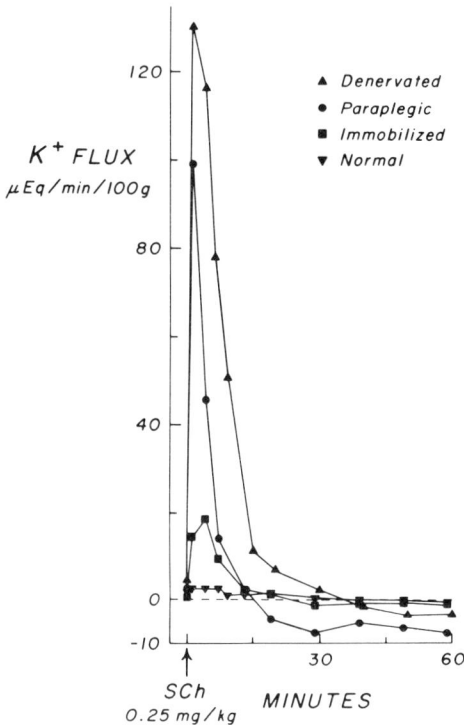

Fig. 18.1 K$^+$ flux following administration of suxamethonium. From Gronert et al.[17]

it follows that this effect becomes prominent 3 days after the denervation. Sensitivity to suxamethonium can continue for 2 years after the injury. Other neurological conditions may also produce a similar hazard. Encephalitis, die back neuropathies and Duchenne-type myopathies are all associated with a risk of K$^+$-induced cardiac arrest when suxamethonium is administered. A similar condition may occur after massive burns, massive muscle damage from crush injuries and after severe infections associated with tissue destruction. Suxamethonium should be avoided in all these conditions.

2 *Malignant hyperpyrexia.* Suxamethonium, especially if combined with halothane, is a potent trigger for this condition in susceptible individuals.

3 *Anaphylactic shock.* Why a compound that is little more than two molecules of ACh should be a trigger for anaphylactic shock is curious but there is ample evidence that this rare condition is more likely to be caused by suxamethonium than any other relaxant.

Is there still a place for suxamethonium?

In spite of all its disadvantages, suxamethonium has unique properties – it produces a rapid, profound, short-lived relaxation.[18] In view of its potential side-effects suxamethonium cannot be justified for routine use for tracheal intubation. Little time is lost if rocuronium is used in its place. For short-lasting procedures mivacurium provides a reasonable alternative to intermittent suxamethonium.

However, for many emergency procedures in patients at risk from aspiration of stomach contents, the ability to obtain perfect intubating conditions in 40 s probably outweighs the slightly increased risk associated with suxamethonium. This is especially true in the elderly and in patients with poor cardiac and respiratory reserve. Suxamethonium is probably the agent of choice in patents with a difficult airway. Not only does it provide the best intubating conditions, but should intubation prove impossible, it is reasonable to anticipate some ventilatory effort within the 3–5-min period that preoxygenation will usually cover. Suxamethonium is widely used for neonates and it has been reported that no adverse effect has been observed in the past in any of the thousands of patients receiving the drug at the Toronto Sick Children's Hospital.[19]

Whilst there is little doubt that the development of new, even faster-onset, non-depolarizing drugs will eventually replace suxamethonium, it should be remembered that in their survey of over 1 million anaesthetics and over 6000 anaesthesia-related deaths, Lunn and Mushin found no higher incidence of death when suxamethonium was used than when other relaxants were preferred.[20]

Pancuronium, vecuronium and rocuronium

The aminosteroid drugs

The demand for a neuromuscular blocking drug that did not cause hypotension led to the development of pancuronium by David Savage at the Organon Laboratories in Scotland. The use of the rigid steroid skeleton for the incorporation of two ACh-like units was suggested by the demonstration of neuromuscular blocking properties of chandonium by Singh and Paul in India in 1972–1974.[21]

Pancuronium found immediate favour as a replacement for tubocurare in cardiac surgery.[22] However, shortly after its introduction, coronary artery surgery displaced valve replacement surgery as the major operation in cardiac surgical practice. Although pancuronium was by no means the ideal drug for patients with coronary artery stenosis, it was so well established that it continued to be the drug that was used in most cardiac surgery centres. Because pancuronium produces an increase in heart rate due to a combination of vagolysis and blockade of the inhibiting neural supply to the cardiac sympathetic system, and as it is also capable of increasing the peripheral systemic resistance due to blockade of noradrenaline reuptake,[23–25] it increases the work of the myocardium.[26] Anaesthetists soon recognized the need to give large doses of analgesics before pancuronium to reduce this effect, which was especially evident after low doses of induction agent. With the advent of the widespread use of β-blockers in patients with coronary artery disease, the side-effects of pancuronium have largely been overcome.

Another major disadvantage of pancuronium is its considerable dependence upon renal excretion for plasma clearance. Although some metabolism and some biliary excretion occur, around 40% of an injected dose is excreted in the urine. It is possible to demonstrate a cumulative effect with successive doses of drug, and delayed recovery of neuro-muscular function is not uncommon. Residual train of four (TOF) >30% in patients in the recovery room has frequently been reported following pancuronium.[27]

In common with all the aminosteroid drugs, the action of pancuronium is markedly prolonged in jaundiced patients – an effect which is believed to be due to the taurocholic acid delaying the hepatic uptake of the drug and a delayed or absent biliary excretion of the drug.

Pancuronium has proved to be an extremely safe drug but the more recently developed aminosteroids have demonstrable advantages. Perhaps the most convincing evidence of this is the study from the San Francisco group, who demonstrated a significantly shorter stay in the recovery room in patients receiving vecuronium rather than pancuronium. Viby Morgensen and coworkers in Copenhagen found a higher incidence of postoperative pulmonary complications in patients receiving pancuronium and alcuronium compared to those receiving atracurium or vecuronium – an effect they attributed to the more complete reversal of the neuro-muscular block.[28] Other workers have also reported more complete rever-sal of residual neuromuscular block when atracurium or vecuronium have been used.[29]

Vecuronium

The cardiovascular side-effects of pancuronium provided the impetus for the development of a 'clean' aminosteroid alternative. Of the many drugs tested, vecuronium, the monotertiary, monoquaternary derivative of pan-curonium, was considered to have the best pharmacological characteristics. It was introduced into anaesthetic practice in 1980.[30,31]

Vecuronium has proved to be the cleanest non-depolarizing drug produced. It has no vagolytic or sympathetic effects in doses up to $60 \times ED_{95}$. Indeed, initially this proved to be the cause of problems, as anaesthetists used to drugs with some vagolytic properties saw the bradycardia produced by opiate and inhalation agents revealed when vecuronium was used. This has led to some anaesthetists accepting that a modest vagolytic effect should not necessarily be considered a disadvanta-geous characteristic of a muscle relaxant. Vecuronium is so lacking in side-effects, even in clinical doses of up to $10 \times ED_{95}$, that it has become the 'gold standard' against which other drugs are compared.

Vecuronium does not produce the rapid onset of an ideal relaxant; in doses $2 \times ED_{95}$ the onset of good relaxation is reliably produced in 2–3 min and its recovery is predictable at 25–30 min. At $3 \times ED_{95}$ there is a slightly more rapid onset of action and a duration of block lasting approximately 50 min. At higher doses the duration of action becomes less predictable.

Like pancuronium, vecuronium is excreted in the urine and bile both as the parent drug and metabolites; however, rather more drug is cleared by non-renal routes. As a result there is only a marginal prolongation of action in anuric patients. The 3 hydroxy derivative of vecuronium has approximately 50% the neuromuscular blocking potency of the parent compound and a longer half-life. Although vecuronium is less cumulative than pancuronium, it has caused reversal problems after being used for more than 48 h either as an infusion or as repeated bolus doses in the intensive care unit.[33-34] The problem has been most commonly observed in children, although there are fewer total case reports in this age group. Three theories have been advanced to explain this problem (which does occur with other drugs, although far less frequently):

1 *Overdose.*[34] It has been suggested that too much drug has been used as few units monitor the return of TOF before giving top-up doses. Whilst this is probably true, it does not explain why it should take 3–4 days to clear the excess drug and allow reversal of the block, nor does it explain why it is less common with other types of relaxant.[36]
2 *Accumulation of metabolites, especially the 3 hydroxy derivative.* Whilst this has been shown to occur to some limited extent, there is no evidence of the presence of a sufficiently high plasma concentration of metabolites in these patients to explain the duration of the paralysis.
3 *A neurotoxicity of the drug.* It is probable that long-term artificial ventilation with or without paralysis can result in changes in the nerves and muscle and acute reversible neuropathies that have been reported in these patients. This effect is seen irrespective of the drug used.

A further possible cause of the difficulty of reversal is that, over days of vecuronium administration, a large proportion of drug remains sequestered in the body in tissues such as the liver, kidney, spleen and cartilage. The sequestered drug will leave the depot sites slowly over the 2 or 3 days following termination of the administration and may provide a constant 'top-up' of the high-affinity sites at the receptors. It is not uncommon to be able to recover only 50% of the dose of vecuronium administered within 6 h of its administration. Although some of this unaccounted-for drug will probably be present in the bowel, it seems inevitable that a considerable depot of drug will also remain in the body.

Whatever the cause, it is probable that other drugs should be used, if possible, for long-term administration or for prolonged infusion in order to provide prolonged muscle paralysis.

Rocuronium

Rocuronium has the most rapid onset of action of any of the non-depolarizing relaxants. In a dose of $2 \times ED_{95}$ the onset time is approximately half that of vecuronium.[37-39] Whilst a rapid onset might be anticipated in view of the reduced potency of the drug, it is still more potent than many drugs with far slower onset. The duration of action in doses up to $4 \times ED_{95}$ is not clinically different from that of a similar dose of vecuronium. Rocuronium is a highly specific agent but in doses over $4 \times ED_{95}$ some vagolysis can be detected.

Like vecuronium, rocuronium is excreted in bile and urine. As the drug lacks a 3 acetyl group, metabolism is likely to be limited; however, the hepatic uptake of this drug appears to be somewhat greater than with vecuronium. Like vecuronium, a considerable proportion of any dose of drug administered remains in the body for a considerable time. Only between 18 and 30% of drug or metabolites has been recovered from urine and bile within 12 h of administration.

Summary of aminosteroid neuromuscular blocking drugs

Rocuronium is the best drug available for easy rapid intubation and its slightly higher cost can be justified on this ground alone. Rocuronium and vecuronium are excellent, highly specific neuromuscular blocking drugs. Their pharmacokinetic profile makes them most suited for administration as large bolus doses or as repeat-dose drugs. As redistribution into the liver and kidneys plays a major part in the plasma clearance of these drugs, it is probable that accumulation will occur if they are used over a prolonged period as once the depot sites are full, only renal and biliary excretion and limited metabolism are available to remove the drug from the body. It is noticeable that after a prolonged infusion of these drugs the time taken for recovery of the TOF is prolonged, whereas the recovery of the TOF after mivacurium infusion is as rapid as after a single ED_{95} bolus dose.

The benzylisoquinolinium drugs

Atracurium

Atracurium was prepared in the laboratories of Strathclyde University in Scotland by Stenlake.[40] The novelty of the drug is that it undergoes spontaneous breakdown to two inactive derivatives in an alkaline pH by a process first described at the turn of the century by Hofmann. Hofmann degeneration produces a tertiary amino byproduct, laudanosine, and an inactive monoquaternary residue. Although it has been suggested that the monoquaternary residue may itself be metabolized in the liver to produce an acrylate, this has only been positively demonstrated to occur with high doses of substrate. Laudanosine has marked central nervous system analeptic effects, although the consequences of this in the concentration found following the routine use of atracurium have been negligible. However, the possibility of producing potentially dangerous by-products or metabolites underscores the problem that may occur when metabolism is the principal method of plasma clearance of drug.

Atracurium is not a pure drug: it can form 10 isomers, but three form the bulk of the commercial preparation – the trans–trans, cis–trans and cis–cis.

Atracurium is also metabolized by plasma cholinesterase.[41] The extent of this process relative to Hofmann degeneration is disputed. Certainly it is a major mode of metabolism in the blood of rodents. The rate of metabolism is fastest for the trans–trans and trans–cis isomers than for the cis–cis isomer. Only a small proportion of the cis–cis isomer is metabolized by cholinesterase. About 10% of an injected dose of atracurium is excreted in the urine.[42]

Although atracurium lacks the high specificity of vecuronium for the neuromuscular junction, it does not produce vagolysis in clinical doses. In doses of $3 \times ED_{95}$ or greater, atracurium may cause hypotension due to histamine release. As a result, atracurium is unsuitable for use in large bolus doses.

The onset of action of atracurium is similar to that of vecuronium but the slower onset cannot be reduced by increasing the dose administered, as it can with vecuronium. However, atracurium is ideally suited for use in prolonged infusion techniques as it does not accumulate in the body and plasma clearance is as rapid after many hours of infusion as at the beginning of the administration.

Atracurium does not rely on hepatic function or renal clearance to reduce the plasma drug concentration and is therefore the drug best suited for use in patients with advanced hepatic disease or anuric patients.[43]

Mivacurium

Many years ago it was suggested that a non-depolarizing drug which was hydrolysed in the plasma-like suxamethonium would have a profile of onset and offset of action like that of suxamethonium. This was based upon the prevalent belief that the onset and offset of block were purely functions of changes in drug plasma concentration. This led to a 20-year programme developing a series of benzylisoquinolinium drugs with an ester bridge between the two quaternary ammonium-carrying groups. Many promising drugs were tested but, until the advent of mivacurium, they all produced unacceptable side-effects, particularly histamine release.

Mivacurium was the first drug to be rapidly hydrolysed by plasma cholinesterase without producing significant side-effects in a $3 \times ED_{95}$ dose. It exists in three principal isomeric forms: trans–trans, cis–cis and trans–cis forms. The minority of the action of the mixture is due to the cis–cis isomer, the only one not to be rapidly hydrolysed by plasma cholinesterase. Virtually all the neuromuscular blocking property of an injected dose of drug resides in the trans–trans and cis–trans isomers, both of which are hydrolysed by plasma cholinesterase at about 80% the rate of suxamethonium (Fig. 18.2). In spite of this, mivacurium is neither a rapid-onset drug nor a drug with a suxamethonium-like duration of action. Indeed, in an ED_{95} dose, its duration of action is similar to an ED_{95} dose of vecuronium.[44] There can be no clearer indication of the fallacy of the original presupposition about the duration of action and plasma drug concentration than the action profile of mivacurium (see Chapter 7).

In spite of the disappointing onset rate, mivacurium in clinical doses – i.e. $2 \times ED_{95}$ – is shorter-acting than an equipotent dose of $2 \times ED_{95}$ of vecuronium and this gives it some advantage where a brief duration of action is a premium requisite. However, against this advantage is the

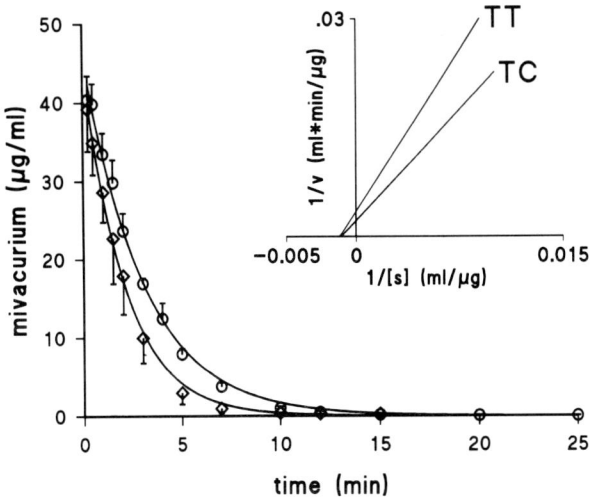

Fig. 18.2 Rate of hydrolysis of mivacurium by human plasma. TT = trans–trans isomers; TC = trans–cis isomer. The small amount of cis–cis isomer is slowly hydrolysed and not shown.

possible disadvantage of a prolongation of action in the presence of a low plasma cholinesterase. In the absence of normal plasma cholinesterase the duration of block may exceed 2 h.

Because mivacurium is not dependent upon renal or hepatic function for its plasma clearance, it would be expected that it would be an ideal, if expensive, drug for continuous infusion techniques and in patients with renal or hepatic failure. However, studies in these patients have shown it to be unpredictable in its duration of action, possibly due to variations in

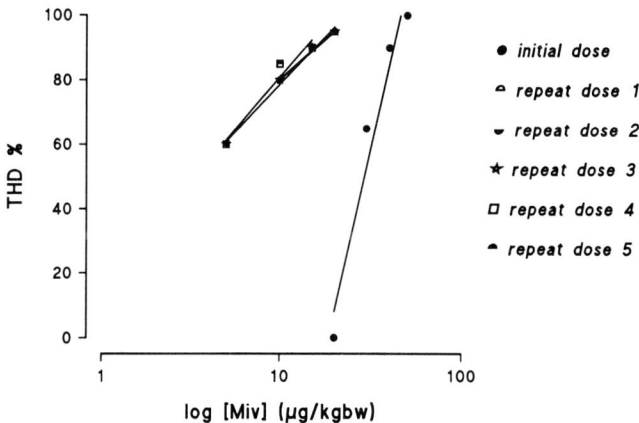

Fig. 18.3 Log dose–response curve of five repeated doses of mivacurium (MiV) administered at 50% recovery of T_1. No evidence of any cumulative effect is seen, although the requirement of top-up doses is approximately 50% of the initial dose. THD = twitch height depression.

plasma cholinesterase levels in these patients. As a result, atracurium remains the agent of choice for patients with serious renal or hepatic disease.[45]

There has been some suggestion of a more prolonged recovery after its long-term use in the intensive care unit, possibly associated with accumulation of the cis–cis isomer or changes in plasma cholinesterase levels in these patients; however, this remains speculative.

Mivacurium is unsuitable for large bolus dose administration as it causes hypotension and flushing due to histamine release. Even after 10 successive doses, the log dose response to mivacurium remains the same as that of the first top-up dose (the ED_{50} of top-up doses are approximately half that of the initial dose; Fig. 18.3). Mivacurium is non-cumulative.

References

1. Feldman SA & Hood JR. Depolarizing neuromuscular block. A presynaptic mechanism? *Acta Anesthesiol Scand* 1994; **38:** 535–541
2. Standaert FG & Adams JE. The actions of succinylcholine on mammalian nerve terminals. *J Pharmacol Exp Ther* 1965; **149:** 113–123
3. Riker WF. (1975) Prejunctional effects of neuromuscular facilitatory drugs. In: *Muscle Relaxants.* Katz RL (ed.). North Holland, pp. 59–102
4. Churchill Davidson HC. Suxamethonium (succinylcholine) and muscle pains. *Br Med J* 1954; **1:** 74–77
5. Watls LR & Dillon JB. Clinical studies of the interaction between *d*-tubocurarine and succinylcholine. *Anesthesiology* 1969; **31:** 39–42
6. Collier C. Suxamethonium pains and fasciculations. *Proc R Soc Med* 1975; **68:** 105–108
7. Baraka A. Self taming of succinylcholine induced fasciculations. *Anesthesiology* 1977; **46:** 292–295
8. Airaksinen NM & Tommisto T. Myoglobinuria after intermittent administration of succinylcholine during halothane anesthesia. *Clin Pharmacol Ther* 1966; **7:** 583
9. Kalow W & Gunn OR. The relationship between the dose of succinylcholine and duration of apnoea in man. *J Pharmacol Exp Ther* 1957; **35:** 339–344
10. Katz RL & Eakins KE. The actions of neuromuscular blocking agents on extraocular muscle and intraocular pressure. *Proc R Soc Med* 1969; **53:** 183–188
11. La Cour D. Rise in intragastric pressure caused by suxamethonium fasciculations. *Acta Anesthesiol Scand* 1969; **13:** 255–310
12. Wylie WD. The use of muscle relaxants and the induction of anaesthesia in patients with a full stomach. *Br J Anaesth* 1963; **35:** 168
13. Mathias JA & Evans Prosser CDG. (1970) An investigation into the site of action of suxamethonium on cardiac rhythm. In: *Progress in Anaesthesiology. Proceedings of the 4th World Congress on Anaesthesiology,* Boulton TB (ed.). Holland: Excerpta Medica
14. Tolmie JD, Joyce TH & Mitchell GD. Succinylcholine danger in burned children. *Anesthesiology* 1967; **28:** 467–469
15. Mazze RI, Escue HM & Houston JB. Hypokolaemia and cardiovascular collapse following administration of succinylcholine to the traumatized patient. *Anesthesiology* 1969; **31:** 540–544
16. Stone WA, Beach TP & Hamleberg W. Succinylcholine danger in spinal cord injured patient. *Anesthesiology* 1970; **32:** 168–172
17. Gronert GA, Lambert EH & Thye RA. The response of denervated skeletal muscle to succinylcholine. *Anesthesiology* 1973; **53:** 13–19
18. Lee C. Suxamethonium in its 5th decade. *Bailliere's Clinical Anaesthesiology* 1994; **8:** 417–440

19. Bevan DR. Succinylcholine. *Can J Anaesth* 1994; **41:** 465–468
20. Lunn JN & Mushin WW. (1982) *Mortality Associated with Anaesthesia.* London: Nuffield Provincial Hospital Trust
21. Sing H & Paul D. Steroids and related studies. Chandonium iodide and other quaternary ammonium steroid analogues. *J Chem Soc Perkin Trans* 1974; **1:** 1475–1479
22. Sellick BA. (1968) Clinical experience of new relaxant – pancuronium bromide. In: *Progress in Anaesthesiology. Proceedings of the 4th World Congress on Anaesthesiology,* Boulton TB (ed.). Holland: Excerpta Medica
23. Duke PC, Fung J & Gartner J. The myocardial effects of pancuronium. *Can Anaesth Soc J* 1975; **22:** 680–682
24. Goat VA & Feldman SA. The effect of non depolarizing muscle relaxants on cholinergic mechanisms in the isolated rabbit heart. *Anaesthesia* 1972; **27:** 143–146
25. Quintana A. Effect of pancuronium bromide on the adrenergic reactivity of the isolated rat vas deferens. *Eur J Pharmacol* 1977; **46:** 275–277
26. Saxena PR & Bonta IL. Mechanism of selective cardiac vagolytic action of pancuronium bromide. Specific blockade of cardiac muscarinic receptors. *Eur J Pharmacol* 1970; **11:** 332–341
27. Beemer GH & Rozenthal P. Post operative neuromuscular function. *Anaesth Intensive Care* 1986; **14:** 41–45
28. Viby Morgensen J, Jorgensen BC & Ording H. Residual curarization in the recovery room. *Anesthesiology* 1979; **50:** 539–541
29. Bevan DR, Smith CE & Donati F. Postoperative neuromuscualr blockade: a comparison between atraccurium, vecuronium and pancuronium. *Anesthesiology* 1988; **32:** 272–276
30. Marshall IG, Agoston S, Booij LDHJ *et al.* Pharmacology of OrgNC45 compared with other non-depolarizing neuromuscular blocking drugs. *Br J Anaesth* 1950; **525:** 11–195
31. Baird WLM, Bowman WC & Kerr WJ. Some actions of ORG NC45 and of edrophonium in anaesthetised cat and man. *Br J Anaesth* 1982; **54:** 375–385
32. Feldman S & Liban JB. Vecuronium – a variable dose technique. *Anaesthesia* 1987; **42:** 199–201
33. Vandenbrom RNG & Wierda JHKH. Pancuronium bromide in the intensive care unit. A case of overdose. *Anesthesiology* 1988; **69:** 996–997
34. Segredo V, Matthy MA, Sharma ML *et al.* Prolonged neuromuscular blockade after long-term administration of vecuronium in 2 critically ill patients. *Anesthesiology* 1990; **72:** 566–570
35. Kunhl-Brady KS, Schreithofer D, Morawetz RF *et al.* (1990) The use of neuromuscular blocking agents in the ICU. In: *Neuromuscular Blocking Agents in Development for Operating Theatre and Intensive Care Unit.* Mitterschiffthater G & Denissen PAF (eds). pp. 103–112
36. Prielipp RC, Courain OS, Scuder PE *et al.* Comparison of infusion requirements and recovery profile of vecuronium and cisatracurium in intensive care unit patients. *Anesth Analg* 1995; **81:** 3–12
37. Mirakhur R, Cooper R, McCarthy G & Elliot D. Comparison of the intubating conditions and some neuromuscular blocking effects following Org 9426 and succinylcholine. *Anesth Analg* 1992; **74:** S210
38. Booik LDJ & Knape HTA. The neuromuscular blocking effect of ORG 9426. *Anaesthesia* 1991; **46:** 341–343
39. Wierda JMKH, de Wit APM, Kuizenga K & Agoston S. Clinical observations on the neuromuscular blocking action of ORG 9426, a new steroidal non depolarizing agents. *Br J Anaesth* 1990; **64:** 521–523
40. Stanlake JB. (1978) Biodegradable neuromuscular blocking agents. In: *Advances in Pharmacology and Therapeutics,* Vol. 13. Oxford: Pergamon, pp. 303–311
41. Stanlake JB & Hughes R. *In vitro* degradation of atracurium in human plasma. *Br J Anaesth* 1987; **59:** 806–810
42. Fahey MR, Rupp SM, Fisher DM *et al.* The pharmacokinetics and pharmacodynamics of atracurium in patients with and without renal failure. *Anesthesiology 1984;* **61:** 699–702

43. Hunter JM, Jones RS & Utting JE. The use of atracurium in patients with no renal function. *Br J Anaesth* 1982; **54:** 1251–1258
44. Savarese JJ, Ali HM, Basta SJ *et al.* The clinical neuromuscular pharmacology of mivacurium chloride (BW1090). *Anesthesiology* 1988; **68:** 723–732
45. Devlin JC, Head-Rapson AG, Parker CJR & Hunter JM. Pharmacodynamics of mivacurium chloride in patients with hepatic cirhosis. *Br J Anaesth* 1993; **78:** 227–231

Index